Tom Ballard, RN, ND

worked in neurology, dermatology, critical care and emergency medicine at the University of Chicago and Virginia Mason Medical Center.

He graduated from Bastyr University in 1982 in naturopathic medicine. Dr. Ballard is founder and medical director of Pure Wellness Centers (www.PureWellnessCenters.com) in Seattle and Renton, Washington which specializes in scientific environmental detoxification and nutritional rejuvenation for the treatment of chronic disease.

Dr. Ballard has written and lectured internationally on such topics as chronic fatigue, kicking the sugar habit, thyroid diagnosis and treatment, anti-aging, inflammation in chronic disease, environmental detoxification, and Green Medicine – treating the cause of disease with natural medicine.

Tom is available for interviews, lectures and teaching.
TomBallardND@gmail.com

D0035348

*"With the Three Wisdoms,
it is as easy as 1-2-3."*

Dedicated to John Bastyr, ND, a curious
mind, perpetual student, and kind soul

Special thanks to
Julie Krauss-Lucas and
hundreds of patients in preparing
this manuscript

Cover photo by
Michael Robbins

Author photo by
Patsy Hilbert

Nutrition-1-2-3

Three proven diet wisdoms for gaining energy, losing weight, and reversing chronic disease

Copyright 2008

Tom Ballard, RN, ND

ISBN 1440483221

EAN-13 9781440483226

Published by
Fresh Press Books
3315 59th Ave. SW
FreshPressBooks@gmail.com

This book has not been evaluated by the Food and Drug Administration. It is not intended to diagnose, treat, cure, or prevent any disease. It is written solely for informational and educational purposes. Please consult your healthcare professional for your specific needs.

Nutrition-1-2-3

The table (of contents) is set with…

SECTION VIII: The Three Wisdoms Join Hands – Bringing it all together

SECTION IX: Little Nibbles – Index of helpful information

Section I

The Appetizers

Chapter 1

Setting the table

Rochelle: Like so many others

Rochelle is intelligent and cares about her health. Several years before her first appointment with me, she read a best-selling health and nutrition book, decided it made sense, and followed it faithfully.

During her time with me I heard a story I've become quite familiar with in my over 25 years in practice. "My energy is entirely unpredictable. Sometimes it's great, and then it's lousy. I have this pain here..." She went on to describe a pain in her abdomen, bloating, premenstrual irritability, muscle aches, and a growing list of allergies. To listen, you would have thought she was sixty years old, not twenty-five.

After two weeks of following the **Nutrition-1-2-3** program, Rochelle felt better. After four months she felt great. One by one her symptoms disappeared. She began to feel so good she decided to go back to school and attempt the graduate program she had been putting off.

However, while she was telling me this good news, she didn't look happy. After she finished, I couldn't help but ask, "Rochelle, I'm glad you're feeling better, but you look, well, angry. Is there something

> *"After two weeks of following the* ***Nutrition-1-2-3*** *program, Rochelle felt better."*

else going on?"

"I am angry. It makes me feel angry every time I think about how I wasted two years of my life and almost ruined my health because of that physician's book. It's a popular book. There must be millions of people doing the same thing. How can we protect ourselves?" Her eyes brimmed with tears. "The newspapers, the health-food stores, TV - they all say different things. I thought I was going to a reliable source of good information."

Rochelle is not alone. It's common for people to feel confused and abused by the contradictory health information thrown at them from different directions. I've had many patients say something like, "I used to watch my diet, but after I read the report that carrots (or whatever) contain a poison, I gave up." Or, "Sometimes I take vitamins, but with all the different opinions, how can you choose?"

Is your health all you want it to be?

Do you have the energy and stamina you need to live the life you want? Is your medicine cabinet empty of prescription and non-prescription medications? Are you free of chronic disease and at a desirable weight? Sadly, most Americans will answer "No" to these questions. More importantly, most people feel powerless to make the necessary changes to improve the quality and quantity of their lives.

Your feelings of powerlessness are all the more distressing because the changes that will dramatically improve your health are very easy once you know the simple formula, the Wisdoms.

Despite what you read about "miracle" drugs and advanced surgical techniques, medical research is very clear that your health is influenced more by simple, every day decisions than any new "medical breakthrough." Yes, wearing seatbelts, not smoking, moderate exercise and eating a healthy diet are well proven to save more lives than any medication. And these "lifestyle" choices are also more powerful than genes at influencing your health.

This book is about the one area of individual health that is often the most confusing to people – what they eat.

What to eat does not need to be bewildering. Once you sort out the sensationalism and fads, it becomes clear that medical research agrees with anthropology and history. Three simple nutritional Wisdoms have withstood the test of time and the scrutiny of nutritional science. To know the Three Wisdoms is to understand the essence of a healthy diet.

A book is born

Nutrition-1-2-3 was born out of the countless conversations I've had with patients like Rochelle. After sharing their bad-diet confessional with me they would often ask, "Isn't there a nutrition book you can recommend?"

To help my patients, I searched bookstores. I found a few good nutrition books on specific topics, such as diabetes and migraines, but no general, basic nutrition books. Certainly people with a specific health problem are more motivated to read books that address their situation, but what about all the people who aren't "sick", but want to feel better? Or, the ones who feel good and want to stay that way? Shouldn't there be a book for them, one that's not a fad-diet book?

If my patients are any indication, there is a need for a concise, easy to read, factual, no-fad, general nutrition book. Frankly, it was embarrassing to admit that with all the research that's been done on healthy nutrition, I could not find any decent books on basic nutrition for the lay person. In a sense, this lack of a good book reinforced the misconception that there is no such thing as good nutrition. No wonder people were giving up and heading for the golden arches.

What can be done for people like Rochelle? Is good nutrition too complicated to be described to the public?

My experience is the opposite. There are simple nutritional principles that can be easily understood. When we separate the hype and hyperbole from science, there are three dietary rules or Wisdoms that have withstood the test of millions of years of evolution and are substantiated by scientific research.

The Three Wisdoms

* **Regularity**
* **Variety**
* **Wholeness**

These are the foundation of healthy eating and healthy eating is the foundation of health. They are the foundation of **Nutrition-1-2-3**, not because they're simple to remember (although I'm glad they are) but because they're tried and true. History and science support their status as Wisdoms of nutrition.

The Three Wisdoms - Regularity, Variety and Wholeness – are easily remembered as **"Regularly eat a Variety of Whole foods."** This manta can make you a nutrition winner at home, in the grocery store and in restaurants.

Historic support for the Three Wisdoms

Historically, we know that hunter-gatherers Regularly ate a Variety of Whole foods. They didn't have a choice. This was the only eating plan available to them. Hunter-gatherers were our ancestors. Their genes were fed by "Regularly eating a Variety of Whole foods." Their genes became our genes.

Humans were hunter-gatherers for 3 million years, but only agriculturalists for 10,000 and industrialists for a mere 250 years. The hunter-gatherer lifestyle influenced our genetic makeup, digestive function, hormonal balances and every other part of our physiology. Starting about 150 years ago with the Chemical Age, synthetic chemicals abruptly entered into our world. More recently, in the past 50 years, fast food and the fast-food lifestyle have further upset the chemical equilibrium that had evolved over millions of years. Even your own great-grandparents did not eat what is now considered the Standard American Diet (SAD). SAD is an appropriate way to describe what most people eat – sad for their health and for the health of the planet.

The hunter-gatherer diet is reflected in the eating habits of contemporary babies who hunt and sample everything (even toes and toys) to discover what they like. They eat a little, rest, and in two to four hours, eat a little more. They don't overeat and they don't miss their feeding time. When they're hungry, they let you know. Research also shows us that babies and children on a natural diet of breast milk and then whole foods will thrive, while those that are fed a SAD diet of baby formulas and fast foods experience high rates of ill health and behavioral problems.

Likewise, adults like Rochelle, who forage too far from the Three Wisdoms often experience chronic illness and premature aging.

"Regularly eat a Variety of Whole foods."

Scientific support for the Three Wisdoms

In addition to the historic record, modern biochemical and nutritional research also supports the Three Wisdoms. Hundreds of scientific studies demonstrate the unhealthy consequences of the Standard American Diet to humans, animals, and the planet. As I will discuss later, these studies uphold the need for returning to a way of eating that more closely resembles that of our genetic ancestors.

Helping you choose the right door

No one can make you eat well. The choice is yours. Many of you, metaphorically speaking, are standing in a kitchen surrounded by mysterious cabinets. Each cabinet door has something behind it. Some things you're sure of, others puzzle you. Unfortunately, much of what you're sure of is incorrect. But you don't need to be confused. The laws, or Wisdoms, of good nutrition are quite clear and easy to understand.

Sadly, the scientific community, educational system, and media have failed to communicate the basic truths of good nutrition. It's no wonder that most people feel confused by contradictory opinions and facts. Often these wrong ideas about nutrition are actually dangerous, creating more ill health. The "low-fat" craze of the last fifty years is an example of a sort of mass-hysteria in which a very narrow bit of scientific information – cholesterol collects in the arteries of some people with heart disease – was extrapolated into a multimillion dollar food and advertising campaign. This book will explain the dangers of "low-fat" and other nutritional fallacies.

You may be a person who looks at the cabinet door marked "Fast-food, delicious and ready to eat" shrugs your shoulders and asks "Why not?" That's not a sign you created, by the way. It was presented to you by the fast-food industry so often that you now believe it. Unfortunately, many people believe the sign that reads, "Health food: yuck!" This belief often develops from eating highly processed "health foods" that are, in truth, expensive, doctored junk foods.

You may have other doors marked with signs such as, "Soda: a fun way to quench your thirst" and "Water: unnecessary and booooooorring" or, "Sugar: for more pep" and, well, fill in the blanks. We all have prearranged notions of what we want in our eating space.

The purpose of this book is to create a context in

which it is easier for you to choose and prepare healthy foods, to rebuild (so to speak) your kitchen with new cabinets filled with healthy, good-tasting foods, founded on solid information. I see my role as the guy who will stand with you in front of the doors and help you see what's behind the labels. Once you understand, you can decide for yourself rather than having the food and beverage industry decide for you.

I know from years of experience that most people are happy to switch from a SAD, or fad, diet to a healthy one after they start feeling the difference. If you're not already convinced that good nutrition will make you healthier, prevent illness and, in some cases, cure disease,

> *"I've witnessed "miracle" cures of incurable diseases for over 25 years. Time and again my patients have seen how simple nutritional changes outperform drug interventions."*

then this book will present you with solid evidence that your choice of food is one of the two most important behaviors for maintaining and repairing health. (The other is exercise).

For those who haven't been exposed to the basics of nutrition, such as what carbohydrates, fats, and proteins are, there are chapters that explain these. Other chapters will show you how easy good eating can be and give you concrete, scientifically verified tools for applying sound nutrition in your daily life. Healthy eating doesn't have to be complicated or confusing if you follow the three simple nutritional Wisdoms that I will explain in detail.

Lastly, this book will briefly review the incredible healing power of diet as applied to most of the common, chronic disease conditions of our age. I've witnessed "miracle" cures of incurable diseases for over 25 years. Time and again my patients have seen how simple nutritional changes outperform drug interventions.

Your life depends on your actions

This book is for doers - people who want to know their diet is scientifically sound and are willing to apply that knowledge with confidence.

Certainly there are nutrition textbooks used in universities worth reading, but I'd suggest you not become too preoccupied by knowing everything. As with most things in life, if you understand and apply the basics, you're way ahead of the game. When you spend your time reading every new book on the market you run the risk of losing sight of the foundation. Wallowing in bookstores also leads some people to postpone applying their knowledge.

Most successful people in business, sports, woodworking, plumbing, or spiritual enlightenment will give you the same advice: You first must understand and apply the basic rules. This book contains the basic rules of nutrition, the Three Wisdoms. I believe by *understanding* and *applying* these rules you can succeed in living a healthier, happier, and more productive life.

Read this book if you are interested in enhancing your life with sound nutrition and if you are like Rochelle - sick of being manipulated by fad diets, bad journalism, and greedy corporations.

How this book is organized

Section I: The Appetizers
Why another nutrition book? This section offers help in jumping off the fad-diet merry-go-round and provides the historic and scientific basis of the Three Wisdoms.

Section II: Ingredients – Beyond the basic food groups
All the basic information you need to know about carbohydrates, proteins, fats, minerals and micronutrients is explained here. If you're not interested in detail or already know this, you can skip this section and proceed into the next.

Section III: The Main Course – The Three Wisdoms
This section explains the Three Wisdoms – Regularity, Variety and Wholeness – and the historic and modern scientific support for their place as the founding pillars of nutritional science.

Section IV: The Three Wisdoms in Action – Shopping, cooking and traveling
How to apply the Three Wisdoms in the grocery store, kitchen, restaurant, and snacking are covered here.

Section V: Three Wisdoms to the Rescue – Treating health problems
Obesity, fatigue, heart disease, skin problems, asthma, diabetes, digestive complaints and food allergies can all be successfully treated by applying the Three Wisdoms.

Section VI: Dinner conversation – Tall tales and myths
Dispelling common nutritional myths such as food combining and milk as the perfect food are discussed here.

Section VII: Aperitifs – Little extras
This section offers additional topics in nutrition and health, from finding a nutritionally-oriented doctor to whether or not you need to take supplements.

Section VIII: The Three Wisdoms Join Hands
This is where we put it all together.

Section IX: Little Nibbles: Index of helpful information

Chapter 2

Nutrition-1-2-3 – Basic questions

If you've ever felt confused about what to eat or frustrated by something you've read regarding nutrition, this book is intended to give you the basic knowledge you need to shop, cook and eat correctly. The following are typical questions my patients ask when we discuss nutritional changes.

Why should I change my eating habits?

If you feel fantastic, sleep well, are pain-free and not taking medications, perhaps what you're eating now is perfect for you. Health is a relative concept. Some people are satisfied with waking up every morning and making it through a non-challenging job. Others want more, sometimes much more. I love working with these people. Everyone should have the opportunity to experience vibrant health – vitality.

Jane's questions

Jane, a 52 year old woman, called me on the suggestion of another patient. She was curious about my services, but wasn't sure she needed any help.

"I don't know if I need to do anything different, I'm very healthy. I only take one medication for my cholesterol."

She was satisfied with her health. Would you be?

My first question to her was, "Why is your cholesterol high?"

"I don't know. My doctor didn't say. I don't eat much fat."

My second question was, "What happened to your estrogen when you artificially lowered your cholesterol with the medication?"

She paused. "What does cholesterol have to do with estrogen?"

"Your liver makes cholesterol and uses it to make estrogen, as well as other hormones. How's you estrogen level?"

"I guess low. I take estrogen."

"So, you're "healthy" but you take two medications – one to lower your cholesterol and one to raise your estrogen?"

"I don't count the estrogen because all women my age take it."

"Not really. Not if their body is making it from cholesterol. But your cholesterol is high and your estrogen low. That's an imbalance. Imbalances in hormones often precede more serious illness. How is your bone density?"

"Good. I don't have osteoporosis, only low normal."

"So, now you've identified another problem, you're only 52 and your bone density is already starting to go down."

"Isn't that normal?"

"Most women in the world have normal bone density, even into old age, except those living in the U.S. and Europe. We can see patterns in your health, even in this limited telephone conversation. Cholesterol effects estrogen. Estrogen affects bones. There may, of course, be other related problems – early skin aging, predisposition to breast cancer, weight gain."

"Yes, of course I'd like to lose some weight."

"This is why they call what I do wholistic medicine. I

refer to it as "Why Medicine" because I'm always asking "Why?" I hope you see that your health is not as good as it could be. The drugs you're taking are only covering up deeper health issues. They may even be contributing to more serious, long-term, health problems."

I've had similar conversations many times. Some people were taught to have limited health expectations. Jane had somehow detached her consciousness about her health from the fact that her weight and cholesterol were high and her estrogen and bone density were low, as if these things weren't really part of her. Would she have believed her car was in good condition if the seat covers were in excellent condition, but the radiator was overheating and the oil was leaking?

Many people are disconnected from their bodies. They don't think of their symptoms as part of who they are. This disconnection is good for the

> *"The two most important things you can do for your health are proper diet and exercise."*

pharmaceutical industry. They're in favor of you taking a pill to stop your knees from hurting, regardless of what that pill is doing to your stomach lining and kidney function. A number of professional athletes have seen their careers cut short by the consequences of ignoring the connections between pain and the rest of their body.

You may not be on any medications. Perhaps you're "healthy" but your energy is low. Or your weight is high. I encourage my patients to take a thorough look at their health and decide if they're living up to their health potential. If not, diet and exercise are the best places to make changes. These are far more likely than drugs to make a difference, and far less likely to cause side effects.

Yes, a natural diet as laid out in **Nutrion-1-2-3** can help restore balance to all the body's systems – hormonal, as well as immune, digestion, nervous system, and skin.

The two most important things you can do for your health are proper diet and exercise. The research is very clear and numerous studies support this. Most drugs are not as powerful or safe as eating well. Diet is even more important than genetics in determining your health. Your two most important daily decisions are what you put in your mouth and whether you take the elevator or the stairs.

While there are a lot of messages out there trying to convince you to eat food that is bad for you, your diet is the one area where you can make a decision every day that will improve your health.

What can I expect from the Three Wisdoms?

The **Nutrition-1-2-3** approach to eating is designed to make you feel invincible in body, mind and spirit. Well, maybe not invincible, that's impossible. However, it will help you get out of bed feeling energetic, with stamina throughout the day, and the physical and mental strength to live an active, productive life. Many people find this approach helps them achieve a more desirable weight.

I've based this book on anthropologic and scientific research. By distilling and organizing the best of what history and science have to offer, I've put together a plan that is relatively easy to implement, yet will yield many positive health results.

Is Nutrition-1-2-3 another fad diet?

No, this is not a fad diet. It's an anti-fad book. Fads come and go. This book is for those who want to know the facts for a lifetime of healthy eating. The principles of **Nutrition-1-2-3** will be useful forever; they've already been around for millions of years. This is not a book that will fall out of fashion.

If you're into fads, there are plenty of other books to

read. I've written this so you can understand and apply sound nutritional principles easily, experience the benefits, and move on with your life. The goal is not to make a diet your life, but to eat a diet that allows you to live a healthy life.

I want to lose weight. Will this book help?

I hear this question a lot, often from women who have damaged their health trying to lose weight. Let's make a firm distinction. Most diet books and weight-loss programs are someone's brainstorm on how to lose weight quickly with minimum effort. These books are not based on any long-term studies or scientific principles, although they make millions of dollars for the authors. They have an almost 100 percent failure rate.

Personally, it makes me angry to see literally hundreds of thousands of people ruining their health and wasting their money on weight-loss diets and products. Yes, they're not just a waste of time and money; they're often deleterious to your health. I write more about this in Chapter 26, Weight Loss for Life.

Nutrition-1-2-3 is for people who are serious about obtaining and maintaining a healthy weight. A healthy weight is the product of healthy living. No shortcuts. No tricks. No "miracle" diets or products. And it especially means no "low fat" or "low calorie" diets.

Is weight-loss difficult? No. Not when you understand the Three Wisdoms.

Will this book help me cure my...?

This book was written as a general guide to optimal nutritional health. It's here to help you evaluate your current diet and give you guidelines on eating the best diet you can. While not a "treatment" book per se, the Three Wisdoms can help you with many health problems.

Section V, Wisdoms to the Rescue, is devoted to

applying the principles of Regularity, Variety and Wholeness to losing weight and overcoming other chronic health problems. These concepts are powerful tools for reducing your risks of diabetes, heart disease, cancer, allergies, digestive and skin problems.

There are plenty of nutrition books for treating specific diseases. Some of these books are excellent and I encourage you to read them if you are dealing with a specific medical condition. I will add, however, that while I support self-help and taking personal responsibility, the advice of a doctor with a solid education in nutrition can be quite valuable. A trained professional will help you avoid mistakes and may save you a lot of time and money. In some cases it can even be dangerous to self-treat.

I understand that finding a competent doctor can be difficult. Chapter 48 provides general guidelines on finding the right doctor for you.

My goal is not to pitch another quick-fix promise and see who buys, but to offer the groundwork for building a diet with staying power. As a basic book founded on sound principles, it can be used for years to come regardless of what "new" scientific research or "breakthroughs" come out. Scientific details in our understanding may be altered in the future, but the basics will not change. The Three Wisdoms have already stood the test of thousands of years of human nutrition.

I've read a lot of self-help books. Why should I read this one?

I believe, and many experts agree, that most popular self-help books are of little or no value. Often they are even harmful. They tend to follow fads and promote "quick-fix" solutions. Many of these books are no more than one person's opinion based on a very limited look at the available research. In general, any book that has 'miracle' or 'revolutionary' in the title or promises you results in a certain number of days, is a fad, a fraud, or a fiction. The Three Wisdoms have stood the test of time and medical scrutiny and will serve you, your children, and future generations to come.

I'm not a scientist. Will I understand this program?

Nutrition-1-2-3 is based on over 25 years of experience with average people from all walks of life. I hope it provides help for you without being too complicated, difficult or confusing.

If you want to know the intricacies of anatomy, physiology, and biochemistry, there are good textbooks available. If you prefer to learn just the basics to be able to make sound decisions, then this book is written for you.

Chapter 3

A morsel of history to nibble on

Predating the dinner table – Hunter-Gatherers

Before we jump into the nuts and bolts of nutrition, let's take a short trip back to where we came from. This journey will give you a strong foundation for future nutritional choices.

Take your mind back in time, way back. Let's remember how our ancestors lived. While many may think of their grandparents, or medieval peoples, or even the early civilizations of Greece and biblical times, I want you to go back further. Before permanent settlements. Before agriculture. Yes, even before buttons.

By far the longest period of human development was in prehistoric times. For most of human existence, before civilization, writing, religion, and most of what we now take for granted materially, we were what are called hunter-gatherers.

Why does it matter what we ate 100,000 years ago? Or even a million? Because your cells remember. Every cell in your body has DNA, enzymes, and other cellular elements that were formed during your ancestors' hunt for food, shelter and water. Your digestive enzymes, your hormone levels, your immune system, your brain and nervous system

– all of you was shaped long ago. It has been said that 99.9% of who we are now was formed during our ancestor's days of roaming for survival.

Let's take a closer look. Even though there is no written history of our early "formative" years, there are first-hand descriptions and anthropological reports on hunter-gatherer communities that lived into historic and even into modern times.

A good place to contemplate life before microwaves, refrigerators, farming, or earthenware vessels is to go to the most native place you can find. A large public park may introduce you to the basics of living like your ancestors. Hopefully there will be a stream for running water, large leaves to act as food containers, roots, berries and wild animals for food, bark for clothing, and enough foliage to protect you from the rain and cold or heat. Just to make it interesting, remember you don't have anything as modern as a steel blade for digging, cutting, scraping and killing. Rocks and sticks are your kitchen appliances.

Is it getting dark and do you feel a little scared? Better sit close to the fire.

Cold? Sorry, you have nothing as light-weight as Polar Fleece. Animal skins are heavy and since there is no Velcro or even buttons, you wrap and tuck and tie. Before there were clothes off the rack there was bark off the tree.

> *"Hunter-gatherers had no domesticated animals, no amber fields of grain, and no 7-11 on the corner. Instead, they ate fresh, organic, unprocessed food."*

Hot? Go naked and know where to find the next oasis.

Depending on what latitude you live at, you may have to spend a considerable part of your energy staying warm or keeping cool. Fruits may grow all year around or only seasonally. Fish may literally jump into your basket or you may have to outrun or outsmart some critter with sharp teeth. Obviously, exercise will not be something you have to find time for; it's how you keep alive. Painting pictographs and telling stories is something you do only in comparably recent times, say 50,000 years ago, and only after you've secured enough food and water.

I highly recommend everyone watch the documentary <u>Nanook of the North</u>. It tells the remarkable story of how one family survived in Alaska - from cutting ice blocks for building igloos to spearing fish and clubbing walruses for food and clothing. It is a true slice of hunter-gatherer life. Nanook and his family's story is all the more moving when you realize that people lived this way for tens of thousands of years. It has only been in the 80 years since the film was made that their way of life has become all but extinct. Similar survival stories existed for most places in the world. Consult the archives of National Geographic Magazine to read about communities that continue to live similarly to their ancient ancestors, but there are few left. Modern civilization has squeezed out native lives.

This basic, no-frills lifestyle is how your ancestors lived. They are where you came from. Their survival nurtured your genes. Some of your ancestors only resembled you superficially. Their skulls were smaller and they had more hair. More recently there were those who, if dressed in contemporary clothes and given a haircut, would go unnoticed in Manhattan.

Hunter-gatherers had no domesticated animals, no amber fields of grain, and no 7-11 on the corner. Instead, they ate fresh, organic, unprocessed food. They had to eat frequently, consuming thousands of calories to keep warm and supply their muscles with energy for foraging and hunting.

The rest of this book will present more details on the implications of your hunter-gatherer background in determining your current state of health. But, let's make one more brief stop. Let's fast-forward from the Paleolithic era to the present.

Pulling your chair up to a contemporary dinner table

Try this exercise. Take out a 12 inch ruler. Imagine each inch is 10,000 years – yes, even older than the food in the back of your freezer. We live at inch 12. At zero, 120,000 years ago, give or take a few thousand, your ancestors controlled fire and regularly cooked with it.

At inch eleven, just one inch ago, in the Cradle of Civilization or the area we now call the Middle East, large scale domestication of animals and grains was taking off. As part of this phenomenal explosion of agriculture, there would soon come – over another five thousand years - irrigation, food storage, social hierarchy, armies, written language, mathematics, governments, and organized religion. We won't delve into all of the changes in society that took place at that time, but I think it is helpful to contemplate the important change in our food supply and eating habits that happened a mere one inch or 10,000 years ago.

"In 125 years we've made what many researchers feel is a dangerous and potentially lethal alteration in diet."

Now, let's divide time up again. Take your ruler and hold your hand over the last two inches so that you only see 10 inches. Each inch now equals 1000 years. We live at inch 0. Ten inches is 10,000 years ago when grains and animals were domesticated and civilization as we know it was beginning. Now look closely at that last inch, from one to zero.

In our exercise, one-half inch ago – or approximately 500 years - the Americas were discovered by Europeans. At one-quarter of an inch ago - 250 years - America was firmly colonized and the American Revolution was about to start. Blood letting was all the rage as a treatment by the leading medical doctors of the time. (Benjamin Rush, MD, one of the signers of the Declaration of Independence, performed the bleeding of George Washington on Washington's deathbed.) During what we now call Colonial times sugar was so precious that rich people kept it under lock and key in specially built cabinets. (You can see them on *Antiques Road Show*).

At one eighth of an inch ago - 125 years - the Civil War was over, most people lived on farms and those were 100 percent organic. Mercury was considered a tonic and was given out like aspirin by MDs. The oil boom was just starting which led to experiments with internal combustion engines, synthetic chemicals (the first was a purple dye) and medicines (aspirin, a synthetic copy of willow bark, was the first). Coca-Cola was one of hundreds of locally-produced patent medicines. Gasoline and cars would soon follow, along with artificial fertilizers and pesticides.

At one-sixteenth of an inch ago – 62.5 years – World War II was raging (with the help of and partially because of oil), someone in your immediate family might have still been alive, and antibiotics were the newly-discovered miracle cure. Farming had switched from horse-power to tractors and from organic to synthetic fertilizers. Locally-produced fresh food was giving way to long-haul trucking. Soon every family would have a car, every city a suburb, and every neighborhood a drive-in. Television and TV dinners were the rage for modern families just as radio and an ice box (with real ice to keep it cool) had been for their grandparents.

How did our dinner table change?

In less than one-quarter of an inch of human civilization – 250 years – the world has rushed from the Industrial Revolution, through the Chemical Revolution, and into the Computer Revolution. In this very short period of time we've gone from the discovery of steel to railroads and cars and spacecraft. In my lifetime, the world has moved from vacuum tubes to transistors to microchips. These jumps in technology have both positive and negative effects. Most people, for example, are happy with labor-saving devices.

But there is one jump that we've experienced in even less time; a change that affects our internal biochemistry, a change so dramatic that we may not survive. In one-eight of an inch - 125 years – we've made what many researchers feel is a dangerous and potentially lethal alteration in diet.

Timeline of Nutrition in History

Hunting and gathering of food for at least 10 million years

Lucy Lived	Homo erectus	Fire
3.2 million BC	1.7million BC	800,000

Homo sapiens	Tools	Agriculture
100,000 BC	70,000 BC	8,000 BC

Herbal Medicine & Acupuncture

Metal working	Old Testament	Rome rules
5,000 BC	1000 BC	200 BC

Jesus
Han Dynasty

Buddhism	Plague kills ½ Europe	Beowulf Classic Pueblo
1AD	500	1000AD

Ming, Mali, Muslim &
Incan Empires

Renaissance in Europe	Bottle & tin cans	Synthetic Chemicals	Sugar = 10-40 lb/yr
1500	1800	1860	1900

More processed foods	USDA: 50% less vit/min in produce
Less organic farming	Several million synthetic chemicals
Pesticides (nerve poisons)	300 lb/yr sugar consumption
1920	2000

Chapter 4

Remembrance of meals past

After tens of thousands of years of fine-tuning the human body to thrive in hunter-gatherer conditions, and another 10,000 years of adapting to primitive agriculture, we leapt from the community organic farm to industrial chemical farming.

We have jumped from eating whole foods to consuming refined, fast foods.

- From zero sugar to nearly 300 pounds a year.
- From zero pesticide exposure to the spreading of tens of thousands of pounds of toxic pesticides on our food yearly.
- From organic, composted soil to artificially fertilized fields.
- From meat, eggs and milk from free-range animals to factory-farmed, high-fat, low-nutrient look-alikes.
- From no chemical additives to additives in almost everything.
- From minimally-tampered whole foods to highly-processed junk foods.

Can our body chemistry make this radical transition and stay healthy?

Many researchers believe we are not making the

transition. The proof is that in this same 125 years, modern industrialized countries have developed epidemic levels of obesity, heart disease, diabetes, arthritis, and cancer – all conditions known to be strongly influenced by diet. At the same time, people who continue eating their traditional foods avoid these modern diseases.

We are adapting to our modern food rather badly. Much evidence suggests that our body chemistry is still dependent on hunter-gatherer eating habits. The weight of nutritional science is telling us that the modern industrialized diet is killing us. Our ancient genes don't know how to handle modern eating.

If each bite of food you eat is a message to your cells, then the message of modern food is an alien language, strange and confusing to our bodies.

It's time to reset our table.

As the first step in setting our healthy table, let's review some fundamental concepts in nutrition. The next section reviews the basics of carbohydrates, proteins, fats, micronutrients, and water.

SECTION II

Ingredients - Beyond the Basic Food Groups

Chapter 5

Food 101 -
What we should have learned in school

We've all seen the food group charts. Food pyramids come and go. And yet many of us are left with questions: What is a protein? How is protein different from fat? What is the difference between fruits and vegetables? How can cheese and fish be in the same category? What category do vegetables fall into?

Sadly, our educational system and the medical community have failed to educate the public on the basics of nutrition. And the media mostly adds to the confusion.

I find it convenient and helpful for my patients to understand that there are five categories of foods:

- **Carbohydrates**
- **Proteins**
- **Fats**
- **Micronutrients (vitamins, minerals)**
- **Water**

Carbohydrates, proteins, and fats are known as macronutrients (macro = large). Micronutrients (micro = small) refers to vitamins, minerals, and other nutrients required in small quantities. Water is also an important "food".

The following chapters explain these categories in everyday language. Once you understand these categories, the rest is simple: apply the Three Wisdoms to eating.

After you become acquainted with the basic food groups it will be simpler to understand the interrelating and overlapping issues. For instance, what about foods that don't strictly belong in one category? What about the quality of the fat you're consuming? Once you understand protein, how much of it do you need each day?

What about beans? They contain both carbohydrate and protein. For the meat eater they may be considered a carbohydrate. For the vegan they're definitely a protein and maybe even the highest protein food in their diet.

I raise these issues not to confuse you, but to emphasize the logic of first understanding the basic food groups. Once you have this knowledge the more complex issues will be easier to understand. Eating well does not require you to know any more than the basic difference between food groups, then applying the Three Wisdoms, which are described in later chapters.

When you understand these basics, you'll know more than most people do about nutrition. Let this knowledge be a tool to empower you.

Chapter 6

Carbohydrates 101 - The energy broker

What is a carbohydrate (or carb)? What's the difference between carbs, starches and sugars? What is the difference in how the body uses them? What do they have to do with diabetes and obesity?

Starch or Complex carbohydrate

The primary fuel or energy sources for the body are carbohydrate foods. A complex carbohydrate, also known as a starch, is made of long chains of carbon atoms. A kernel of wheat, corn, or rice is mostly complex carbohydrate. Beans, potatoes and squash are also common examples. Vegetables or fruits contain a mix of starches and sugars. A sugar is a simple, short, chain of carbons.

A way to visualize a carb is to imagine a chain. Each link of the chain is a carbon molecule known as a sugar. Another name for a carbohydrate is polysaccharide (many sugars). The longer the chain, the more complex it is. The shorter it is, the simpler and thus the term "**simple carbohydrate**." A chain of carbons that has been milled or ground into shorter pieces is a **refined carbohydrate**. Its original long structure has been shortened.

- **Carbohydrates:**
    - o **Simple: sugars**
    - o **Complex: starches**

Of course, all of these carbohydrate foods also contain a percentage of protein, fats, vitamins and minerals. No food is only one group, but most will contain a predominance of starch, protein, or fat. Nuts, such as almonds, are a good example of a food that contains protein, carbs and fat. Meat, likewise, is mostly protein, but also contains fat and small amounts of starch.

It is important to remember that most vegetables and fruits are mostly carbohydrates. So, when you're trying to make a decision as to what to eat for the carbohydrate portion of your meal, don't just think of grains and potatoes, but also broccoli, salad greens, peas, beans and all other vegetables and fruits. The exception is avocados, which are primarily fat.

Sugar and glucose

When a long chain of carbon atoms is split into smaller pieces, it just so happens that these short chains taste sweet. These small carbs are known as sugars. The sweeter the food, such as a ripe banana, the more of the starch has been converted, or broken down, into its individual sugar pieces.

In nature, natural sugars are produced by enzymes breaking chains of carbohydrates into shorter sweet chains. An unripe apple, for instance, has more long-chain carbs. As it matures, enzymes convert or break the carbs into sugars. The sweetness of any fruit, vegetable, bean or grain will depend on the amount of sugars.

Sugars are "**simple**" or short carbohydrates. They are made of single or double carbon atoms. There are several types of sugars depending on which molecules are combined. Sucrose, or table sugar, is composed of two simple sugars - **glucose** (also known as dextrose) and **fructose**. Because there are two sugars, it can also be called a **disaccharide** (two sugars). Sucrose is 99.9 percent "pure", meaning it has been stripped of all other nutrients. Sugar is usually made from the refining of sugar cane or sugar beets – thus comes the term "**refined sugar**."

Lactose is a sugar found in milk. It contains equal parts of glucose and **galactose** which is another simple one carbon sugar.

The process of **refining** or extracting sugar from cane or beets requires several steps. An early step is cooking the cane or sugar beet into syrup. As the syrup becomes more concentrated, sugar crystallizes and separates out. Molasses is the remaining syrup after the sugar crystallization has occurred. Brown sugar is sucrose which still has some of the molasses mixed in. Turbinado sugar is a slightly less refined table sugar – 95 percent refined. So-called "raw" sugar is 96 percent pure. I say so-called because it is not raw, only cooked less than table sugar.

Sugar striptease

Refining removes almost all other nutrition elements from a sugar. **Protein, fats, fiber, vitamins, and minerals are stripped away.** Despite claims to the contrary, turbinado and raw sugar do not contain enough vitamins or minerals to contribute meaningfully to your health.

Some foods, such as fruits, are high in the sugars glucose and fructose. These are the same two sugars that make table sugar. However, the difference between the sugar in an apple and table sugar is that the apple also has water, fiber, vitamins, minerals, and some complex carbohydrates. These make the apple more nutritious and slow the breakdown and release of sugar into your bloodstream. This slow-release of sugar is a key element in keeping you healthy. More on this can be found in Chapter 32 which discusses blood sugar regulation and diabetes.

Refining carbohydrates

As mentioned above, through mechanical and chemical processing the long chains of carbons that make up a starch are broken into shorter pieces to form a refined carbohydrate. When a kernel of wheat is harvested, it is a complex carbohydrate or starch. As it is milled, ground, and bleached, the carbon chains are broken into shorter chains. During the refining process, protein, fiber, vitamins and minerals are removed or destroyed. This refining process could literally turn wheat into sugar if carried out far enough.

The most common examples of refined carbohydrates are refined wheat, rice and corn. High-fructose corn syrup is the most commonly used sweetener. This extract of fructose from corn is used in many processed foods and sodas.

> *"Protein, fats, fiber, vitamins, and minerals are stripped away."*

For millions of years, through our ancestors' time as hunter-gatherers, complex carbohydrates were broken down slowly within the body by chewing and the enzymatic action of saliva and pancreatic enzymes.

Refined carbohydrates, because they require less chewing and natural digestive breakdown, are absorbed through the intestinal lining and released into the bloodstream faster than a complex carbohydrate. When you eat refined carbs, or sweets, you bypass the normal digestive processes and speedily release sugar into your blood.

Eating refined carbs is like burning paper instead of logs. Food processing turns whole foods, the logs, into paper. What results is a quick burn rather than a sustained heat.

In the past one hundred years, food processing plants have been predigesting carbs, so to speak, outside your body. When you eat this refined product it floods your cells with sugar at a faster rate than they have the evolution to handle. This rush of sugar into the bloodstream and cells causes unhealthy changes in blood sugar, hormones, and fat levels.

Calories in carbohydrates

Each gram of sugar contains four calories. A calorie is simply a unit for measuring heat or energy. When your body "burns" or metabolizes foods, the resulting energy is measured in units of calories. Calories are to energy as pounds are to weight.

A lot of emphasis has been placed on "low calorie" dieting in the past 50 years. One of my goals is to convince you that "low calorie" diets and calorie counting are usually unnecessary and often counterproductive to healthy eating and weight management.

Chapter 7

Carbohydrates 202 -
Fuels that steal, fuels of steel

Consider this chapter extra credit if you want to know more about how carbohydrates fuel our bodies.

Insulin and Glucagon

There are two important hormones that regulate blood levels of glucose. You've probably heard of insulin, but may not know exactly how it works. Glucagon is as important as insulin, but is less well known.

Basically, insulin and glucagon are hormones that control sugar passage in and out of cells. When I refer to "cells" I mean all of the cells that make up your body. Insulin and glucagon control the glucose or energy levels throughout your entire body - muscles, kidneys, brain, skin, etcetera.

Let's say you've just eaten peas which are mostly a carbohydrate. During digestion the carbohydrate is broken down into sugar which then passes through your intestinal walls and into your blood stream. So far, so good. That sugar is circulating as potential energy for cells.

However, for sugar to give you energy it must pass out of the blood and into a cell. Sugar does nothing in the blood. It is inside the cell where sugar is turned into energy.

The energy produced inside the cell is used to produce heat, repair tissues, manufacture hormones, and is integral to every other function that keeps you alive.

Insulin is a transporter of sugar. It is a hormone produced in the pancreas that circulates in the blood and acts as a carrier for transporting glucose into the cell. It is like a forklift that scoops up the sugar molecules and carries them from the blood and into the cell. Once inside the cell, the sugar can either be burned for energy or, if the cell is overloaded, it will be stored for later use as fat.

Glucagon is another pancreatic hormone but it counteracts the action of insulin. It moves sugar out of the cell and back into the blood so it can travel to where it's needed. For instance, when you are exercising, glucagon signals the liver cells to release glucose into the blood where it flows to the working muscles for energy.

Ideally, insulin and glucagon are working in balance to keep the sugar moving in and out of the cells as needed. Think of insulin and glucagon as the traffic controllers for sugar.

When this balance is disrupted, diabetes (high blood sugar) or hypoglycemia (low blood sugar) may result.

Now you understand more about glucose control than most people, including some doctors.

Sugar: Thief of life

As explained above, sugar has little nutritional value in it except calories. All the extras, like protein, fiber, vitamins and minerals were removed in purifying it. Why does this matter? **Digestion, transport and utilization of calories requires protein, fiber, vitamins and minerals**. If your foods aren't supplying you with the necessary nutrients, your body will steal these from other places. Therefore, sugar is a thief; it is a "food" that steals nutrients from your body.

For instance, chromium, zinc, manganese, magnesium and several B-vitamins are necessary for the transportation of sugar into the cell. Insulin does not work alone. The forklift needs helpers. Insulin needs these **vitamin and mineral "cofactors"** to assist in its work of transporting glucose into the cell.

When sugar comes into the body without supportive vitamins and minerals, such as with eating candy and excessive refined carbohydrates, the body must steal these cofactors from tissue stores. Therefore, sugar is an anti-food. It robs the body of nutrients. I call sugar and refined carbohydrates "**Foods that Steal**".

> *"Ideally, insulin and glucagon are working in balance to keep the sugar moving in and out of the cells as needed. Think of insulin and glucagon as the traffic controllers for sugar."*

On the other hand, if you're eating a complex carbohydrate, complete with its other food factors, it will be broken down into simple sugars, and it contains the vitamins and minerals required for transporting the glucose into your cells. Complex carbohydrates bring along insulin's cofactors. The forklift has the helpers it needs to do its work.

How could sugar be bad for me?

Sometimes when I'm counseling patients on the evils of sugar, they look at me like I'm a little crazy and ask, "But don't we need to eat sugar for energy?"

My answer is "No. Absolutely not. Quite the opposite. People lived healthy lives for thousands of years without refined sugar. "

It was first shown as early as 1806 and confirmed in many experiments that people and animals die faster on sugar than they would if eating nothing.

What the body needs, and what it evolved over thousands of years to need, are calories in the form of complex carbohydrates containing other nutritional elements, not refined, lifeless, sugar.

Historic legacy of sugar

The sugar trade was integral to the slave trade in America. Africans were taken to the West Indies where they were sold to sugar plantation owners. The sugar, molasses and rum that these slaves produced were shipped to Europe and the Americas where they were sold or traded for furs and other goods. The enslavement and murder of 20 million Africans was part of the economic impact of the sugar trade. The historian William Duffy once wrote, "No other product has so profoundly influenced the political history of the Western World as has sugar." Sugar, a highly-refined "drug" with enormous economic importance, has obvious parallels to opium and its trade in the East.

Environmental costs of sugar

The West Indies sugar trade flourished until Barbados, the British Indies and, later, Cuban agricultural lands were exhausted by repeated planting and burning cycles. Walter Reed, the famous doctor whose name now adorns a prestigious hospital in Washington D.C., gained his reputation by discovering a vaccine against yellow fever which was killing Cuban sugar cane workers. This is another example of how medical advances often coincide with economic interests.

Today, millions of acres of land that could be growing vegetables for undernourished people in Latin American, Africa and Asia are instead growing sugarcane and beets. Sugar is a "hard currency" crop, used to create wealth for large landowners and to pay back World Bank loans. The low-paid workers sweat for long hours under dangerous conditions for meager wages.

The United States, in order to insure its sugar self-reliance, has a domestic sugar cane industry that requires the drainage and environmental destruction of portions of the Florida Everglades.

What about substituting artificial sweeteners?

Forget their appealing names - Sweet-n-Low, NutraSweet - and remember what they are: artificial.

How does your body know what to do with something that is not part of the natural body chemistry? After millions of years, your body has developed ways of dealing with most natural substances. Carbohydrates and natural sugars are recognized and dealt with appropriately. Artificial sweeteners are strange creatures from another planet. Philosophically that's enough to keep me away from them.

In addition, the scientific research into the safety of these products does not put my doubts to rest. Numerous reports of migraines, disorientation and ringing in the ears have been documented. People with a history of epilepsy are cautioned against using aspartame because of the possibility that it may trigger seizures. People with a certain genetic condition, phenylketonuria, do not metabolize aspartame well.

No long-term studies have been completed on these products. They are in progress on a huge, unsuspecting population of diet-pop drinkers. Some critics claim that aspartame was approved by the FDA commissioner over the objections of his own board of inquiry. Later this commissioner was hired by the makers of NutraSweet.

> *"No long-term studies have been completed on these products. They are in progress on a huge, unsuspecting population of diet-pop drinkers."*

There are also no long-term studies showing these products help people lose weight, which is the primary reason people use them. In fact, some studies have found that artificial sweeteners actually cause people to gain weight! This is probably because it encourages sweet-seeking behavior.

There is simply no compelling reason to use artificial sweeteners and too many questions about their safety to relegate them to the "No, I don't care to be a Guinea pig" category.

Carbohydrate choices

Not all carbohydrates are created equal. Some react quite differently in our bodies than others. You may have seen charts showing the rating of carbs by Glycemic Index or Glycemic Load. These can be useful tools, especially for weight loss and diabetic control.

Glycemic Index

Glycemic Index (GI) is a tool for differentiating the effects of carbs on your blood sugar. A low glycemic food produces a low rise in blood sugar and a high glycemic food produces an elevated rise in blood sugar.

Why does the GI matter? Because when the blood sugar goes up quickly, as when eating high glycemic foods, your body triggers the release of insulin. As insulin levels go up, you're more susceptible to diabetes, heart disease, obesity and inflammation.

The following chart illustrates the difference.

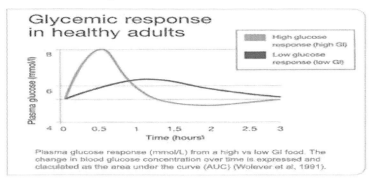

Plasma glucose response (mmol/L) from a high vs low GI food. The change in blood glucose concentration over time is expressed and claculated as the area under the curve (AUC) (Wolever et al, 1991).

Note the difference in the curves. Radical swings during the high glucose response (high GI) are unhealthy. The smoother low glucose response (low GI) is more compatible with health.

Low GI foods help control weight gain, insulin levels, diabetes and cholesterol. They slowly release sugar into the cells for a more sustained release of energy. The only advantage of high glycemic foods is for quickly restoring energy stores after extreme exercise.

For the most part, examples of high and low glycemic foods are obvious. Sugar, fruits and refined carbohydrates have high glycemic indexes. Whole grains, vegetables and nuts have low glycemic indexes. Refined grains, like oatmeal and white flour, tend to fall into the medium to high range.

Glycemic Load

Glycemic load (GL) is a refinement of the GI ranking system. The weakness of the GI system is that it doesn't take into account the quality of the carbohydrates in the diet. For instance, a peach and a piece of bread might be rated the same in spite of their obvious quality differences.

GL makes up for this weakness of the GI ranking by multiplying the GI by the number of grams of the food divided by 100.

A comparison of GI with GL differences is seen clearly in a food like watermelon. Watermelon is rated high in GI but only moderate in GL because the actual amount of sugar one consumes in watermelon is small as it is mostly water.

Beyond Glycemic Index and Glycemic Load

While GI and GL can be useful tools, especially for those who are following a strict diabetic diet, for most of us there is an easier and less cumbersome way of sorting out which carbohydrates to avoid and which to include. Besides, it's not much fun to always be remembering lists or calculating sums. We want to eat and enjoy, not sit and worry.

Another job for the Three Wisdoms!

If you're Regularly eating a Variety of Whole foods, the GI and GL are taken care of without having to think about them. Variety means you're not just eating one food. Whole means you're not eating refined foods with a high GI.

If you only have a bag of grapes for lunch, then you're eating only a high GI, high GL food. This is not a good idea if you're trying to lose weight, reduce your cholesterol level or control your diabetes. But, if you combine a small number of grapes with a piece of cheese then the GI of the grapes doesn't matter. The GI of your entire meal is low. This is the magic of Variety. Your snack consisted of a carb – grapes - with fat and protein – cheese. Isn't this why we like peanut butter on our bananas? It adds Variety and balance to a snack.

Carbohydrate checklist

Here is a simple checklist you can use while you're getting started with the Three Wisdoms program. These will help you choose the best carbs. Once you've practiced these a few times it will become second nature.

When choosing a carb, ask yourself these questions:

- Does it contain mostly complex or mostly simple starches?
- Fruits are mostly simple starches. Beans, grains and vegetables, including potatoes, will be mostly complex. Sweetness is a good test: the sweeter the taste, the simpler the carbs. Refined carbs, such as white flour products, are mostly simple.
- How much protein and how many other vital nutrients does it contain?

A fruit is mostly simple carbohydrates, yet it contains water, fiber and many vitamins and minerals as compared to candy which is also simple but without the other food factors. Millet is mostly complex carbs, but also contains a considerable amount of protein. Potatoes contain a little protein but are mostly starches and sugars. Both millet and potatoes are full of vitamins, fiber and minerals.

So, do you choose millet or potatoes?

This is a trick question because it depends on the rest of the meal and what else you've eaten that day. If you had millet for breakfast, the Variety rule suggests you go for the potatoes. On the other hand, if there is no other source of protein in the meal, then you're better off with the millet because it contains more protein.

Too complicated? Once you've memorized the mantra, **"Regularly eat a Variety of Whole foods"** you can make food choices in seconds.

Better quality sugars?

When I'm educating patients about the evils of sugar, I'm often asked, "What about fructose?" or "Doesn't honey have vitamins in it?"

The following is a brief description of most of the common sweeteners. I do not recommend eating any concentrated sweet more than as an occasional treat.

The similarity of these products, that is, their high sugar content, far outweighs any small differences they possess in the amount of vitamins.

Corn syrup:

This is made from corn which has been treated with sulfuric or hydrochloric acid, then neutralized and bleached with other chemicals, becoming glucose and water with every nutrient removed. Often sucrose is added to increase sweetness. It's very cheap and used in many processed foods.

Fructose:

Most fructose is made by adding several industrial enzymes to corn syrup to produce sucrose. This is then broken down into glucose and fructose, the two molecules that comprise sucrose. Fructose can also be made from refined cane or beet sugar which has the glucose-fructose bond broken. It may be made from natural sources such as fruits and vegetables, but this is rare as this process is very expensive. Even fructose from "natural" sources is a highly refined industrial product.

Contrary to popular belief and advertising from "health foods", fructose may be the unhealthiest sweetener of all.

Honey:

Blossom nectar, which is mainly sucrose, is broken into the monosaccharides (mono=one, therefore one-sugar) glucose and fructose by bees. Honey contains 80 percent sugar. The other 20% is mostly water. The honey is then heated to kill bacteria and viruses. "Natural" honey is heated under lower temperatures (between 100 and 145 degrees F°) in an effort to preserve enzymes, vitamins and pollen. Raw honey is not heated or is only heated to 95-105 degrees. Yes, honey contains traces of vitamins and minerals, but in bee-size quantities.

Maple syrup:

100 percent pure Grade A maple syrup is 65 percent sucrose. The rest is water and traces of vitamins and minerals. Lesser grades have lower sugar content which the distributor often makes up for by adding refined sugar. It takes 40 gallons of sap from sugar maple trees to make one gallon of maple syrup. It is the most expensive sweetener.

Malt:

Cereal grains are processed into syrup by enzymatic action. Malt is made from sprouted barley which is dried and powdered to be used in malting other grains. The malt is mixed with barley, rice, corn or wheat and heated, which converts the starches to sugar. The sugar contained in malt syrup is mainly maltose which is less than half as sweet as sucrose.

Barley malt syrup:
As the name says (a rare instance of truth in advertising) it is a sweetener made from barley. It is less sweet than both molasses and honey because it is higher in complex carbohydrates. Because of this, it enters the bloodstream more slowly. It also contains trace minerals and B-vitamins in very small amounts.

Brown Rice Syrup:
It is primarily a complex carbohydrate. It does contain some B-vitamins and trace minerals, but not as many as barley malt syrup.

Sorghum molasses:
This is refined from a plant related to millet. The stalks are crushed and the sweet syrup released is cooked and clarified into a dark syrup rich in minerals such as potassium, iron, calcium and the B-vitamins. It is about 65 percent sucrose.

Blackstrap and Barbados molasses:
These are the juices extracted from sugarcane on the way to making table sugar. They contain mostly simple carbohydrates, with some water and trace amounts of minerals.

Brown Sugar:
Brown sugar is just white sugar that has had some molasses mixed in to add coloring.

Date sugar:
Date sugar is made from dehydrated dates and is high in fiber and rich in vitamins and minerals. It's difficult to use in cooking because it does not dissolve in liquids. It's also expensive.

Agave syrup:
Highly refined from cactus juice. Often contains as much fructose as refined corn syrup.

Changing your sweet tooth into a healthy tooth

If you are addicted to sweets, you may find this difficult to believe, but you can lose your sweet tooth. Yes, it will be a challenge for the first few weeks or months, but you can lose your addiction. I will cover this more in the chapters on weight control and blood sugar. But, I assure you, sweet cravings are a biochemical as well as a psychological problem. When you change your biochemistry with the Three Wisdoms, your desire for sweets will diminish and become controllable. Please don't think of yourself as a "weak" person who can't control his or her urges. You have learned a behavior that has upset your body's chemistry. By re-balancing your chemistry you can gain control of your sweet desires.

Carbohydrate lesson

The historic record and modern science agree that natural, complex carbohydrates from whole grains, beans, nuts, roots, vegetables, and fruits are the healthiest forms of these foods. When refined into simple carbohydrates and sugar they are associated with nutritional deficiencies and health problems.

For more information see also chapter 26: Weight loss for Life and Chapter 32: Diabetes and Blood Sugar.

Chapter 8

Protein 101 - Structure and function of life

Protein is necessary for both the structural and functional components of health. It provides structural support in the form of muscles, tendons, ligaments and other connective tissues. It is also the core of many hormones such as insulin and growth hormone and pain-modulating endorphins. Proteins are also necessary for immune function and blood clotting. Enzymes are proteins that break down foods, help synthesize and repair tissues, and produce energy. Proteins affect fat levels, such as cholesterol, by attaching to them and moving them out of circulation.

Protein composition

Protein is made from chains of nitrogen atoms. Short pieces of proteins are known as amino acids. There are 20 different amino acids which, when combined in various ways, make up tens of thousands of different proteins.

Amino Acids

Of the 20 amino acids, eight are termed "essential." It is essential that we eat them because our body doesn't make them. The eight essential amino acids are (this is extra credit): lysine, valine, phenylalanine, tryptophan, isoleucine, lucine, methionine and threonine.

Individuals who are eating a Variety of protein foods generally have no trouble meeting their need for essential amino acids. Vegetarians and people with chronic disease or digestive problems may become deficient in certain amino acids if they're not careful about their eating habits.

Calories in protein

A gram of protein contains four calories.

Other components of protein foods

Just like starches, most protein foods also contain other nutrients. Meats also contain fats in varying amounts and very small amounts of carbohydrates. Beans combine protein with starch and tiny amounts of fat. Cheeses have protein and fat, and some contain carbs in the form of lactose. Nuts have protein, carbohydrates and fat.

Standard recommendations: How much protein?

One of the questions I'm asked most regarding nutrition is, "How much protein should I eat?"

It's important to note that protein is not stored in the body like fat is. It must be replenished each day or protein will be scavenged from muscles. This means you must eat enough protein daily to meet your needs. Protein starvation results in the body breaking down muscle and other body proteins – not a good idea.

The standard, nutrition-textbook answer to this question is one-quarter to one-half gram per pound of body weight. A 150 pound person then will require approximately 38 to 75 grams. Biochemical individuality, digestive function, activity levels, heredity and many other factors affect how much protein you need.

Some authors and the RDA split the difference and

recommend 0.75 grams of protein per kilogram of body weight. At this rate a 150 pound person would require 52.5 grams. A 138 pound person would require 50 grams. Apparently, the FDA does not believe in any variables other than weight.

Children, because they are growing, have higher recommended levels:

- A newborn up to five months of age - 2.2 gram of protein per kilogram. That's 1 gram of protein per pound of body weight. This high requirement is because the newborn is growing at such a rapid rate.

- One to 6 years of age - 1.2 grams of protein per kilogram of body weight.

- 7 to 14 years of age – 1 gram of protein per kilogram of weight or one-half gram per pound

- Over 14 years – The same as adults.

Conditions that increase the need for protein include pregnancy, lactation, chronic illness and mal-absorption which are all common conditions in modern society.

Some studies claim that the typical U.S. diet supplies more than these recommendations. Men in these studies typically take in 75 percent more than the RDA and women 35 percent more. Is this a problem, or are the standard recommendations too low?

What is a high protein diet?

The last 15 years has seen an increased popularity of high-protein diets. Dr. Atkins wrote several best-selling weight-loss books and has advocates all over the world. Variations on his theme have emerged. The South Beach Diet was quite popular a few years ago.

Critics of Atkins point to the amount of saturated fat that comes with this level of protein. They believe it is unhealthy for the heart. Excessive protein also places a burden on the kidneys and has been shown to drain calcium from the bones. A March 2007 study published in the Journal of the American Medical Association (JAMA), comparing various weight-loss diets absolved the Atkins diet from any harmful effects and rated it better than the commonly prescribed low-fat diet, the Zone Diet and the South Beach Diet. I emphasize, however, that the differences in these diets were small and the study only lasted one year.

The criticisms over high-protein, high-fat intake have proven to be mainly theoretical. Actual cases of harm have not been demonstrated. In fact, as in the JAMA study, high-protein, high-fat diets often lead to lower levels of cholesterol.

In my opinion, part of the popularity of the high-protein diet is that it is a backlash against the high-carbohydrate diet that has been popular among mainstream nutritionists since the 1970s. The high-carb diet has been a health disaster. Many researchers now feel that the low-fat, high-carb diet has contributed to the increasing rates of obesity, diabetes and heart disease seen in the past few decades. Because of this, the pendulum has swung in the opposite direction to relatively low carb, higher protein diets. My experience has been that blood-glucose sensitive people often do better by raising their protein levels. If they maintain this for a few months, along with other healthy lifestyle changes, they can often go back to a more moderate protein intake.

Thankfully, it appears the popularity of the high-carb diet has run its course. We know it has created more health problems than it has solved. On the other hand, the high-protein diet is more expensive and difficult for most people to maintain. Our tongue's built-in craving for carbs is difficult to overcome.

Moderately High-Protein Diets

In thinking about how our early ancestors ate, remember that they were not eating much in the way of grains. There was no structured agriculture. Their carbohydrates came from roots, nuts, fruits and vegetables.

Some anthropologists believe that hunter-gatherers consumed high amounts – 45 to 65 percent of calories - from animal foods. Further, researchers believe that only 14 percent of our ancestors derived more than half of their calories from plant foods. Obviously there were climate and seasonal variations. Natives of the north ate a very high protein and fat diet and were healthy and not overweight. Equatorial peoples ate more carbohydrates. One estimation for the "average" hunter-gatherer from societies worldwide is that proteins comprised 19 to 35 percent and carbohydrates 22 to 40 percent of their total calories. These numbers are higher than RDA recommendations and lower than Atkins. They are more in line with the Zone and South Beach Diets, as well as current research.

Comparing you to your early ancestors raises some complications.

Do you work as hard as hunter-gatherers? Generally not.

Do you rely on your own production of body heat as much as early peoples? Most of us live indoors and have central heating as well as insulated clothing.

These two factors reduce our need for calories. What about our ratios of carbs, protein and fats? Should we be eating the same amount of protein as the "average" hunter-gatherer? It's not an easy question to answer, but it seems a good place to start.

Determining your need for protein

Given what we know – that our ancestors ate relatively high protein diets and that these diets are shown to help with obesity, diabetes and other modern health concerns - I recommend that my patients embark on a little experiment to determine their ideal protein intake.

1. Determining your current protein intake

- Step one: Write down everything you eat for a week.
- Step two: Total up the amount of protein you take in for the week. (Nibble B in section IX at the end of the book contains a list of common whole foods and the amount of protein in these foods. Packaged foods will have the protein content listed on the label.)
- Step Three: Divide your weekly total by seven. This gives you your average daily protein intake.

2. How you feel with your current amount of protein?

The signs of deficient protein include loss of weight, excess weight (if starches are high in the diet), a high body fat percentage, low energy, poor wound healing, frequent infections such as colds, poor muscle tone and water retention (edema). Blood protein levels are not a reliable measure of adequacy unless you suffer a profound deficiency and protein stores have been exhausted.

I find that patients who complain of blood sugar problems including periodic fatigue, irritability, sugar cravings, depression and loss of concentration are often protein deficient. Read more about this in Chapter 32: Diabetes, Hypoglycemia and Blood Sugar.

3. How does your protein intake compare with established norms?

Are you eating somewhere between one-quarter to one half gram of protein per pound of body weight?

4. Adjust your protein intake to fit your need

If you're not feeling as well as you think you should and if your protein intake is lower than one half gram per pound, then increase your protein for a month and see how you feel.

Let's say your weight is high for your height and you are eating, on average, only one-quarter gram of protein per pound of body weight. My suggestion would be to double your protein intake to one-half gram per pound for four weeks.

Another example would be the person who has low blood sugar swings throughout the day but is eating one-half gram of protein per pound of body weight. These people are probably getting plenty of protein, but may be eating most of it at dinner rather than distributing their intake throughout the day. Timing of protein intake has profound influences on energy, cravings and blood sugar swings, so before increasing your total, read the following section on timing meals.

Confounding factor – meal timing

Meal timing (and especially protein timing) is another factor in determining the ideal amount of protein to eat.

It's not uncommon to find people who are eating the "right" amount of protein, but seventy-five percent of their protein is eaten with dinner and none with breakfast. Numerous studies show this a prescription for gaining weight. The most successful dieters eat breakfast.

Chapter 15 talks about Regularity and meal timing in detail. For now I will just say that to accurately determine your individual requirement for protein you need to be eating protein at each meal and you must eat breakfast.

In the Nutrition-1-2-3 program your goal is to **"Regularly eat a Variety of Whole foods."** I emphasize that every meal and snack should contain some protein.

Generally I aim for a moderate protein intake. If you're having blood sugar problems or need to lose weight you may go a little higher, but not to the Atkins high-protein level. I keep my hypoglycemic patients on a moderately high protein diet for 3 to 12 months, until their blood sugar is stable, then I let them experiment with less protein. Some people can lower their protein without problems. Others start to gain weight and have their symptoms recur. This is especially true in what are called "grain sensitive" people. In this condition, the person maintains a healthy weight and energy level on meat, dairy and vegetable protein, but on grains, especially wheat, they gain weight.

Timing Example

For instance, let's use a person who is 5'5" and weighs 175 pounds or 79.5 kilograms. This theoretical person is overweight. Let's say she is already exercising daily. When we had her keep track of her protein intake for a week she averaged 50 grams a day. That's not a bad amount as it is within the range commonly recommended for her weight. One-half gram of protein per pound of body weight would equal 80 (rounded off) grams. Let's say she is already eating breakfast with protein and eats Regular meals throughout the day.

So, even though she's doing a lot of healthy things, clearly it's not working. She would feel better, look better and have a better chance of living longer if she lost weight. Let's also assume she doesn't have any health problems such as low thyroid function.

Given that she's exercising and eating a reasonable amount of protein and eating breakfast, what can we recommend for her?

I would suggest she increase her protein to the upper level of what is commonly recommended – 80 grams per day. I would emphasize that she spread out her protein intake so that she's eating 20 grams at each meal and 10 grams at each of two snacks. In one month we would reevaluate her body composition by taking her weight, measurements and percentage of body fat. Rarely would this person not lose weight with this strategy.

Obviously we're assuming a best-case scenario. This person is healthy, exercising and eating breakfast. In reality it is hard to find a person like this.

When to recalculate protein intake

If you are purposely losing weight or gaining weight (because you want to increase muscle mass) with your new level of protein intake you will need to periodically recalculate your protein need. As a general rule, recalculate with each 15 to 20 pound change in weight. As you can imagine, losing 15 pounds will reduce your need for protein.

For people who aren't changing weight but need a periodic reminder, I suggest recalculating protein needs at the beginning of each year and measuring your protein intake for one week. This acts as a healthy reminder and often counterbalances the excessive intake of carbohydrates of the holiday season. It's a healthy way to start the New Year.

Protein individuality

The above calculations are based on averages and may not apply to you. There are many differences in how efficient individuals are at digesting, absorbing, and utilizing proteins. Some people's livers are better at converting proteins. We know that some individuals do well on a lower intake of protein, while others require more. What's important is your individual need.

Please don't use this statement or the argument of biochemical individuality to ignore these guidelines because you believe yourself to be an exception. The only way to prove you are an exception is to have a thorough health assessment and by taking an honest look at your health. If you are healthy, really healthy, you are probably getting enough protein. But if you have any health problems such as an unhealthy weight loss or gain, a high percent of body fat, recurrent infections, depression, joint pain, fatigue, depression, rising blood lipids, diabetes or other chronic problems, then your protein intake needs to be valuated along with the rest of your health.

I'd like to emphasize the body fat measurement. It is entirely possible for you to be at a "normal" weight, yet be high in body fat. The only way to know is to measure. Remember, if your percentage of fat is high, then your percentage of muscle (protein) will be low – this is a prescription for ill health. Doctors who are knowledgeable about weight-loss will have scales that measure your fat for you. Cigarette smokers who control their weight by smoking often fall into the category of normal weight but high fat percentage. This makes them less healthy than the overweight person who has a relatively lower fat percentage.

> *"In my experience, most people have no idea of how much protein they're taking in. Calculating your theoretical protein needs and following that recommendation for a few weeks can be a real eye-opener – and an energy and mood lifter."*

Animal verses plant protein

This is a complicated issue bringing in anthropology, history, genetics, ethics and biochemical individuality.

There are many good arguments for a vegetarian diet, and I encourage my patients to eat 30 to 50 percent of their protein from non-meat sources.

Large scale population studies favor the health benefits of vegetable-based proteins.

Environmentally, it has been estimated that reducing meat production by 10 percent would provide enough vegetable-based food to feed 60 million people. The argument is that grains are much more efficiently used as human food than as animal food. It takes 8 to 12 pounds of grains to produce a pound of meat.

On the other hand, I've seen many patients over the years that don't do well as strict vegetarians. Some fail because they don't take the time to educate themselves or because they don't apply that knowledge in the kitchen. Often they want to eat like everyone else - lots of carbs, processed foods and sweets - but leave out the meat. This is a recipe for disaster.

To be a healthy vegetarian you have to restructure how you shop, prepare foods, and eat. While excessive carbs are unhealthy for anyone, they're even worse for vegetarians whose diet is already weighed in favor of carbs. The rule of Variety is especially applicable to vegetarians. They should never eat carbs alone. They're already getting plenty of carbs in two of their protein sources – beans and grains. Eating eggs and dairy helps tremendously because of their protein content. Vegetables alone supply little protein. All grains are mostly starches, but millet, amaranth and quinoa are higher in protein than other grains, approaching the content of beans. Vegetarians must be very careful about taking in starchy foods such as potatoes and corn unless they are very active physically.

Variety can be a problem for vegetarians and especially for vegans who don't eat eggs or dairy. Vegetarians sometimes overly rely on dairy products. I've known vegans who only know one bean - soy. Nuts and seeds can be helpful additions to these diets as well as the dozens of other beans out there.

Hard as it may be to believe, some vegetarians eat too much overly-processed food. They buy fake meat substitutes that are littered with preservatives and, not to be dismissed, excessive packaging. If you're going to be a healthy vegetarian, get to know a big Variety of Whole beans and grains and learn how to cook them.

I've also treated many vegetarians who rarely eat vegetables. Strange as this may sound, these individuals consume large amounts of grains, but few green, red and yellow vegetables. This usually causes a slow decline in health.

People with allergies or food sensitivities to grains have a difficult time staying healthy. Becoming a vegetarian compounds the problem. This is no trivial matter since estimates are that as many as one in five people are grain sensitive. This means that they are not extracting all the nutrients from the grain and are also triggering inflammation. Food-sensitivity inflammation occurs commonly in the digestive system, lungs, skin, joints, and brain. Symptoms from diarrhea to depression have been reported. (See Chapter 36: When Good Food Turns Against You.)

To me there is only one reason to be a vegetarian - personal ethics. If the idea of killing animals is repugnant to you, then be a vegetarian. Some people believe that eating meat is inherently unhealthy. History and science disagree. The health arguments against meat only apply to factory-raised animals. If you're going to eat meat, eat healthy, organic, grass-fed meat. The same goes for dairy and eggs. The environmental arguments against meat don't apply to free-range ranching in which the cows, sheep, chickens and pigs are integrated into a multilayered farm environment.

Other arguments against meat eating, such as our ancestors were vegetarians or our bodies won't digest it, are inaccurate and based on poor science. Our ancestors ate meat when it was available. There are no human cultures or animals that strictly avoid meat. Even "vegetarian" animals eat protein-rich bugs. Our teeth and digestive systems work very effectively for an omnivorous (vegetable and meat) diet. Mostly vegetarian animals have longer digestive tracts. Meat eaters tend to have shorter digestive tracts. Your digestive system is ideally evolved to eat everything (within reason).

If you personally have a problem digesting meat, you're probably not digesting a good many other things as well. The solution is not to avoid meat, but to get your digestion fixed. Digestion is fundamental to your health. Find a physician who can help you.

> **Nutritional deficiencies sometimes associated with vegetarianism include:**
>
> - Protein
> - Calcium
> - Zinc
> - Iron
> - Copper
> - Manganese
> - Vitamin D
> - B vitamins, especially B12

I'm not saying all vegetarians have these deficiencies, only that they need to be monitored. Dietary adjustments may be necessary to avoid any deficiencies.

I do agree that most Americans eat too much meat and not enough vegetable protein. However, strict vegetarianism and especially veganism (no meat or diary) can make it difficult to function optimally in a demanding world. Again, I go back to the basics: measure your current protein intake for two weeks. If that level is keeping you healthy and happy, great. If not, reevaluate.

If you're considering becoming a vegetarian, I suggest you do so gradually. First, improve your current diet. Switch to organic foods, increase your vegetable intake, and cut out refined foods. Also, see a wholistic practitioner for a good health exam to address any health problems you may be having. An excellent resource on vegetarianism, veganism, and raw foods is www.beyondvegetarianism.com.

Eggs: To eat or not to eat?

When discussing protein with patients, the question of eggs often arises. The egg question is symptomatic of a medical system gone crazy. Eggs have been demonized for the last few decades because of their cholesterol content. This has done more harm than good.

Attributes of eggs

- They are an excellent source of high-quality protein.
- They are relatively inexpensive.
- They are easy to cook.
- They can be cooked in many ways, including mixed in with other foods in ways that make the eggs unrecognizable.
- Their low price and ease of cooking makes them especially appealing to older people who otherwise often do not consume enough calories or protein.
- They contain lecithin, a natural compound that helps break down fats.

Problems with eggs

Eggs are maligned primarily for their cholesterol content. Let me make a few quick points.

- For most people, there is not a direct correlation between eating cholesterol and having high blood cholesterol. In fact, over the past thirty years cholesterol consumption has gone down, yet blood cholesterol and heart disease rates have gone up. More on this in Chapters 9 and 33, on fats and heart disease.
- A certain amount of cholesterol is necessary for body function. The liver manufactures cholesterol for use by cells and hormones.
- Even the conservative American Heart Association has changed their tune and now states that seven eggs a

week is fine.
- Organic, free-range eggs are lower in cholesterol and higher in healthy omega-3 oils than factory eggs. Big agriculture has ruined eggs as it has all other foods. Buy organic and free-range eggs.
- High temperature frying (as done in most restaurants) has a negative effect on egg protein and fat. To prevent this, poach, hard boil or fry with olive oil over low heat.

Maligning natural, healthy foods

An organic egg is a good, wholesome food with many healthy attributes and few or no drawbacks (except for those with egg allergies). Why was it targeted as a "no-no" food? Why are people encouraged to eat high-carbohydrate foods instead – especially since it is known that excess carbs are turned into body fat and are associated with ill health more so than the simple egg?

I could propose a conspiracy, but the reason is more likely just because the medical industry is so far removed from anything natural and under-educated about nutrition that it is apt to send simple, incomplete messages to the public. Cholesterol deposits in arteries therefore stop eating cholesterol. This is a simplistic interpretation of a much more complex process involving inflammation in the arteries, other chemical mediators, nutrient deficiencies, and untold issues we don't yet understand.

Another factor that derailed our diets onto the no eggs, low-fat fad was the national panic over heart disease that began in the 1950s. Heart disease is a serious problem. The response from the medical-industrial-complex has been drugs (statins), high-tech surgical techniques, and illogical dietary recommendations. What they ignored was the fact that heart disease didn't start with the eating of eggs, but with the modern era of processed foods. Heart disease rates were extremely low in 1900 and have risen along with the intake of processed foods.

If you like eggs then enjoy them. Select fresh, locally grown, organic or free-range eggs from contented chickens and rotate them through your diet.

Protein all the way

Protein is your friend and only wants to be treated like one. The take home message is to Regularly eat a Variety of Whole (fresh, organic, unprocessed) protein.

Start by finding out how much you're currently eating and compare that to your weight, percentage of body fat, and how you feel. Periodically recalculate your intake based on how your health and what your weight is doing.

Chapter 9

Fats 101 -
Good, bad and vital

With all of the bad rap they've gotten, it's sometimes hard to convince people that some fat is good, even vital. You can't live without fat. Fats are an integral part of every cell of your body.

The old saying, "You are what you eat" is especially true of fats. If you eat bad fats, they become part of every cell and tissue of your body. Scientists now have a better understanding about the complexity of fats in our body and the differences between good and bad fats.

Although you wouldn't know it to read the diet suggestions in popular magazines and from many MDs, science has gone way beyond the "low-fat" advice of the past few decades.

Basic Fat Concepts

Certain fats are called "essential fatty acids," (EFAs) because your body cannot manufacture them. It is essential they're eaten in your diet. The much-maligned fat cholesterol is so important for your health that the liver actually manufactures it. Cholesterol becomes the building-block of hormones and other vital elements. Fats and oils are important for the health of your heart, blood vessels, nervous system, immune system, and skin.

Calories in fats

Fats are higher in calories than proteins and starches. A gram of fat is equal to nine calories. However, I caution you not to presume more calories equals bad.

What are fats?

(Also see illustrations at end of this chapter.)

You usually know them when you see them, but knowing a little chemistry goes a long way in clearing up confusion. Just so we're all talking about the same thing, here is some basic terminology.

Lipids

These are waxy, oily or fat-like substances that repel water and combine with similar chemicals. This is why butterfat floats to the top of the milk and why oil and vinegar must be remixed each time you use them. Fats and water don't mix. Fats and fats do mix.

Lipids are made of a chain of carbon atoms. Common lipids are cholesterol, fat, oils, waxes, phospholipids (a major component of cell membranes made up of phosphorus plus lipids), and the fat-soluble vitamins - A, D, E, K, and carotene. Getting the idea that there are good fats?

Fat

Fat in the body is often in the form of a triglyceride. A triglyceride consists of three fat molecules (thus "tri-") held together by a glycerol (a type of glucose). Imagine a microscopic E, with the upright line being glycerol and the three lateral arms being strings of fats. The name of the triglyceride depends on the type and length of the fat arms. More on this later.

Fat is a concentrated energy source for the body. Fats also carry flavors in foods and help create a feeling of satiety (feeling full). Fat gets into your body because you eat it, but it is so important that your body can also manufacture it from carbohydrates or protein. The fact that excessive carbohydrates can raise blood lipids and cause you to gain weight is one of the reasons why high carb/low fat diets have been such a health disaster.

Fats are classified as saturated or unsaturated.

Saturated Fat

Saturated fats are solid at room temperature. They are called "saturated" because every carbon atom in the chain has a hydrogen atom attached (see diagram). These hydrogen atoms "fill up" the bonding sites and block other atoms from attaching. Think of the back-bone of the fat, the carbon atoms, as being a row of parking spaces. When the fat is saturated, a car (hydrogen) occupies every space.

Typical saturated fats are found in animal products and certain vegetable oils such as coconut and palm oils. The saturation makes them thicker or more solid.

Many people equate "saturated" with "bad." But saturated fats are necessary for life and serve many useful purposes. Like most other things in health, it's a matter of balance. You want some, but not too many, saturated fats. Also, cholesterol is not the same as saturation. They're two different animals, both serving important functions.

Methyl Group H_3C Omega end	Carbon Chain CH_2 Variable length	Carboxyl Group -COOH

<----------------- Fatty ------------><----- Acid ----->

Why is this a saturated fat? Because every carbon (C) is saturated with hydrogen (H), blocking oxygen from attaching.

One advantage of saturated fats is that because all the parking spaces are filled, it is difficult for oxygen to attach and break it down. We all know the result of fats that have been broken down by oxygen – rancidity. Therefore, saturated fats from animal sources and coconut and palm oils are called "stable", meaning they don't break down readily at room or even at moderately high temperatures. This makes them excellent for cooking.

Unsaturated fat

An unsaturated fat does not contain enough hydrogen atoms to "fill" its bond sites. Some of the parking spaces are empty. Therefore it is unsaturated or not full. Most vegetable oils and fish oils are unsaturated. Unsaturated fats are liquid at room temperature and are usually referred to as oils.

Since hydrogen (a car, in our analogy) does not occupy each parking space, oils are susceptible to oxygen attack. Oxygen can attach (park in) the empty bond sites and break down the oil causing rancidity. In this instance the oxygen molecules are known as "free-radicals." This attack is referred to as oxidative (oxygen) or free-radical damage. You've heard of antioxidants. They are compounds that stop the oxidation of fats.

Free-radicals are not always bad. For instance, they are useful for killing invading bacteria. But too many can cause cell and tissue damage. Many disease states have high levels of free radicals – cancer, diabetes, arthritis, Alzheimer's. Indeed, most inflammatory states are triggered by free-radicals. Again I repeat, as with most systems of the body, the key to health is balance.

Unsaturated fats are considered "unstable" in that they will break down at room temperature and are especially vulnerable to oxygen damage when heated. That is, they "oxidize" easily. This makes them poor choices as cooking oils. When you eat an oxidized oil, it is taken into your body and will trigger oxidative damage in your cells. Yes, cooking with soy, corn, and safflower oil makes you vulnerable to oxidative damage.

There are two types of unsaturated fats or oils, described below.

Monounsaturated:

This is an oil in which one pair of hydrogen atoms is missing. All the parking spaces are full of cars except one. One = mono. It only has two open spaces for an oxygen molecule to park in. Olive and avocado oils are examples. With only one parking space available for oxygen, these oils are fairly stable at room temperature.

Another name for monounsaturated oils is oleic oils.

Monounsaturated

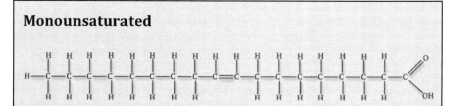

Oleic Acid: Commonly found in olive oil.

Omega end (CH_3) followed by 17 carbons.

Oleic Acid is an 18 carbon molecule. Note at the 9th carbon there is a double bond (=). This makes oleic acid an omega-9 fatty acid (numbering always starts from the left (omega) position). Double bonds open up space for oxygen to move in and attach to carbon atoms. This makes monounsaturated fats less stable than saturated fats, but more stable than polyunsaturated fats.

These oils tend to be less solid than saturated fats at room temperature, but more solid than polyunsaturated fats (described below). This is why olive oil that is refrigerated will be solid, but left out at room temperature will be liquid.

Polyunsaturated:

These oils have many (poly-) empty hydrogen sites, or free parking spaces, for oxygen to attach. With all these unsaturated sites, polyunsaturated oils are the most susceptible to rancidity. To slow down rancidity, they can be kept refrigerated or have vitamin E, or other antioxidants, added for protection.

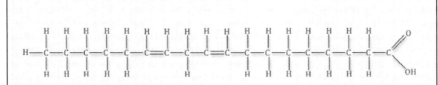

Linoleic Acid (LA):

An 18 carbon fatty acid with the first double bond (=) at the 6th carbon making it an omega-6 fatty acid. It has two double bonds making it a **polyunsaturated oil.**

Polyunsaturated fatty acids (PUFAs) are abundant in soy, corn and most vegetable oils. PUFAs are also Essential Fatty Acids (EFAs) in that your body does not manufacture them, so you must eat them. They are liquid at room temperature.

How do you like your fries?

Here's a question for you: Is it better to eat fried foods cooked in saturated or unsaturated oils? I hope you were able to answer "saturated" and are wary of products that claim superiority because they're fried in unsaturated vegetable oils – the oils most likely to cause oxidative damage.

Essential Fatty Acids (EFAs)

Essential, in terms of nutrition, means you can't live without getting it through your diet. If the body needs a nutrient, but doesn't manufacture it, it is termed essential. It is essential to eat EFAs, so don't leave home without them.

There are two essential fatty acids and they are both polyunsaturated fats.

Linoleic Acid

Linoleic Acid (LA) is a chain of 18 carbon atoms and belongs to the omega-6 family of fatty acids. This family name simply means that the first double bond (where two hydrogen atoms are missing from parking spaces) is in the sixth position. Again with the parking lot analogy: LA is a central strip of 18 concrete blocks (carbon atoms), each with a potential parking space on each side. But, since there are two double bonds, the first after the sixth carbon, some of the parking spaces are missing hydrogen.

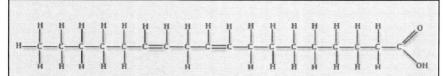

Linoleic Acid (LA):

An 18 carbon fatty acid with the first double bond (=) at the 6th carbon making it an omega-6 fatty acid. It has two double bonds making it polyunsaturated.

Linoleic Acid (LA) converts to **pro-inflammatory** molecules:
- Prostaglandin E-2 (PGE-2)
- Thromboxane -2 (TXA-2)
- Leukotienes

Linoleic acid is a major component in cell membranes and helps keep cells flexible. Flexibility helps them change shape, squeeze into small space and decreases their fragility; they bend before they break.

Linoleic acid can be converted into (pardon my language, there are no common names for these compounds) **Arachidonic Acid** (AA) which in turn becomes **Prostaglandins** (PGE-2) and **Thromboxanes** (TXA-2). PGE-2 and TXA-2 are hormone-like chemicals that trigger many essential bodily functions including blood clotting, pain, inflammation and smooth muscle contraction. Arachidonic acid can also be converted to the more potent **Leukotrienes**, powerful agents of inflammation. Leukotrienes are 10,000 times more potent than histamine in causing allergic sensitivity including bronchial spasms in asthma. One of the concerns about eating excessive amounts of animal proteins is that they contain more aracidonic acid than vegetable proteins.

Common signs and symptoms of an omega-6 fat imbalance include bumps on the back of the upper arms, dry hair, hair loss, dry skin, eczema, brittle nails, and slow wound healing.

Alpha Linolenic Acid (ALA)

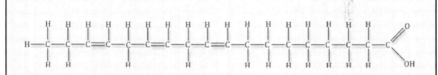

Alpha-linolenic Acid (ALA):
An 18 carbon fatty acid with the first double bond (=) at the 3rd carbon making it an omega-3 fatty acid. It has 3 double bonds.

ALA contains 18 carbon atoms, like LA, but has its first double bond after the third carbon atom. This gives it a classification as an omega-3 fatty acid.

ALA is high in fish, pumpkin and flax seed oils. Fresh vegetables, organic meat and dairy also contain omega-3 oils. Note, it is the ORGANIC varieties of meat and dairy that contain these healthy oils.

Common signs and symptoms of an omega-3 fat imbalance are numbness and tingling of the extremities, impaired immune system function, frequent infections, mood swings, depression, senile dementia, and post-viral fatigue.

Omega-3 oils lower blood cholesterol and reduce the risk of clot formation in the blood vessels. ALA is converted to **Eicosapentanoic acid (EPA)**. (At last, something you might recognize!)

EPA

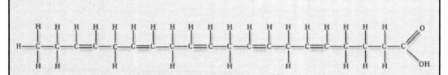

Eicosapentaenoic Acid (EPA)
An 18 carbon molecule with the first double bond at the 3rd carbon making it an omega-3 fatty acid. Note there are 5 double bonds making EPA more susceptible to oxygen attack. **EPA** converts to **anti-inflammatory:**
- Prostaglandin-2 series (PGE-3)
- Thromboxane -3 (TXA-3)

Eicosapentanoic acid (EPA) is a modification of ALA and is also an omega-3 oil. It is high in fish and shellfish. EPA can be converted to prostaglandin PGE-3 and thromboxane TXA-3. These are called the prostaglandin and thromboxane-3 (three) series.

PGE-3 and TXA-3 reduce clotting, pain and inflammation. They balance the PGE-2 and TXA-2 series that increase clotting, pain and inflammation. Balances like this are a recurrent theme in animal and human chemistry. Balance is compatible with health. Imbalance leads to disease. In this case, too much of the "two-series prostaglandins" leads to more allergy, inflammation, clotting and pain. Sound familiar? This imbalance is very common.

EPA deficiency can result in inflammation and muscle contraction anywhere in the body - digestive system, urinary system, muscles, brain. For optimal health, omega-3 and -6 oils should be kept in balance. This keeps the pro- and anti-inflammatory responses in balance.

The heart-healthy effects of omega-3 oils are so well established that they have recently become available by prescription (for a much higher price than over-the-counter brands of the same fish oil).

Because fish oil is polyunsaturated it is susceptible to rancidity. Quality brands do not taste overly fishy. Taste your brand by biting open the capsule. If it tastes sharp or strong, discard the bottle. Bad oil is worse than none. Also, make sure that your fish oil is free of mercury and other contaminants such as heavy metals, PCB's, and dioxins.

DHA

Docosahexaenoic Acid (DHA) is another omega-3 oil that is also high in fish oils.

Some EPA's are converted in the body to DHA which is the longest and most highly unsaturated fatty acid in membranes. Because of this, it is the PUFA most likely to undergo oxidative damage. So, while it is extremely good for you, it is very susceptible to oxidation.

The highest levels of DHA in the body are found in the brain, nerves, retina, and testes.

These two elements - a long chain of highly unsaturated fat and high levels in brain and nerve - may lead you to the same conclusion that many researchers have verified: the health of nerve and brain tissue requires high levels of DHA and lots of antioxidants to keep oxygen from attaching to those empty parking spaces. Or, you might say it is very good to have a lot of empty parking spaces as long as you can keep them from being damaged.

DHA is considered critical for membrane fluidity and permeability. When it is part of a cell's membrane, it allows for proper hormone and nerve receptor function. In other words, it's vital for communications between cells. And it's critical in allowing nutrients to pass into cells and waste to move out.

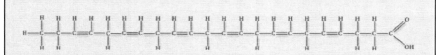

Docosahexaenoic Acid (DHA)
A 22 carbon molecule with the first double bond at the 3rd position making this also an omega-3 fatty acid. Note there are 5 double bonds to be attacked by oxygen.

DHA is high in the brain and nervous system. We are all fat heads!

Low DHA causes reduced membrane fluidity which alters hormone regulation, among other things. Deficiency causes the effects of estrogen, progesterone and angiotensin (a hormone that raises blood pressure) to be exaggerated. Insulin (blood sugar regulation) and serotonin (mood) effects are diminished when DHA is low.

Low DHA causes poor cellular communication and regulation and contributes to the following diseases: breast cancer, PMS, depression, senility, hypertension and insulin-resistant diabetes.

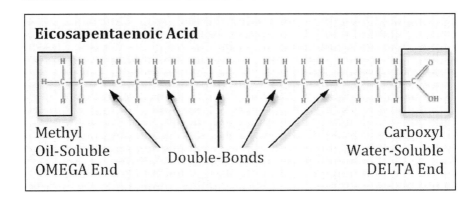

Eicosapentaenoic Acid

Methyl
Oil-Soluble
OMEGA End

Double-Bonds

Carboxyl
Water-Soluble
DELTA End

The Anatomy of Melancholy, by Robert Burton and published in 1652, recommends a diet rich in borage oil and fish for depression. The author didn't know what DHA was, but knew the effects. If only more of the medical establishment understood basic nutritional biochemistry.

When DHA supplementation is given, there is a dramatic increase in the number of synaptic vesicles. Or, in plain English, more nerves fire. Monkeys on low omega-3 oils show hyperactivity, increased aggressive and anti-social behavior. Low DHA in humans causes similar problems. A cure for the common teenager?

Everyday oils

In real life, few oils are purely one type or another. Usually foods and oils contain a combination of different types of fat. For instance, canola oil is classified as polyunsaturated because that is its primary constituent, but it also contains high amounts of monounsaturated fats. Olive oil is 72% monounsaturated, while avocado oil is 69% and almond oil is 68% monounsaturated. Polyunsaturated fats make up the remaining portions. Traditionally people ate a Variety of fats, often changing with the weather and location.

Functions of Fat

Forget the anti-fat hype. Fats and oils are essential for life. They are needed for energy, cell structure and function, and proper brain and nerve activity.

Fats = Energy

People tend to have negative perceptions of fat. For instance: fat = calories = weight gain. But, remember, calories are a measure of energy. I like to think: fat = energy.

Yes, fat is stored energy. Fat is the largest storehouse of unused energy. Calories, when metabolized in cells, are burned to produce energy. Fat stores more than twice as many calories of ENERGY than carbohydrates or proteins. The body usually only maintains a small amount of carbohydrate in the liver for quick energy. Most of the protein is busy doing useful work or providing structure.

It's fat that sits, like a charged battery, waiting to be switched on. (Actually, it's much more dynamic, constantly turning over and being mobilized into different useful molecules, but "charged battery" is a useful analogy.)

If your muscles need more energy to complete a race or climb the office stairs, fat may be called upon. If the liver's detoxification processes are being taxed by a prescription drug or environmental toxin, then fat stores are ready to supply more energy. Every function of the body, from pumping blood, to digesting food, repairing the skinned knee and contemplating the universe, requires energy. Fat is there to make sure the calories are available to get the work done.

Yes, some people have too much stored energy. They need help mobilizing their fat into useful work. But excess fat is not the problem, it is a symptom. Symptoms should not be sucked out by surgeons, but listened to.

Fats = Cell structure and function

Fat is the core structure of every cell in the body. Cell membranes are made of phospholipids - a combination of phosphorus and fat. It's the fat that allows the membrane to be solid enough to hold the cell together, yet flexible enough to mold into different shapes. Think of an egg out of its shell. A thin membrane holds the white and yolk together.

The liquid quality of the fat also allows molecules and compounds to pass in and out of the cell. Oxygen, for instance, diffuses through the cell membrane into the cell. At the same time waste products can pass easily out of the cell to be taken up by the blood and removed.

The function of the cell is affected by the quality of the fats that are eaten. If you eat predominantly saturated and hydrogenated fats, your cell membranes will contain more of these. If you eat healthy omega-3 oils, your membranes will be made primarily of these oils. The difference is that a predominantly omega-3 membrane will be more elastic, less likely to break, and will allow for better flow of nutrients and information in and out of the cell.

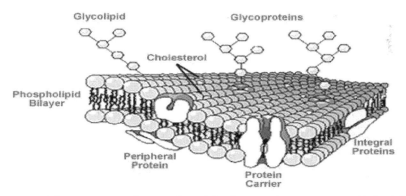

All aspects of your health depend on your cells' ability to keep the traffic of chemicals and electrical impulses moving smoothly. Fat is a major contributor to that flow of good health.

Fats = Brain and nerve function

The brain is composed of about 70 percent fat. Myelin, which speeds nerve transmission, is made of fat. Yes, we are all "fat heads." The quality of the fats we eat directly affects the functioning of the brain and nervous system. DHA, an omega-3 oil, is the ideal fat for brain and nerve function. Yes, be a "fat head", but be a healthy one.

Note in the following illustration that a fatty myelin sheath surrounds the nerve axon. This allows for faster conduction of nerve impulses. Multiple sclerosis is a disease in which the myelin is damaged.

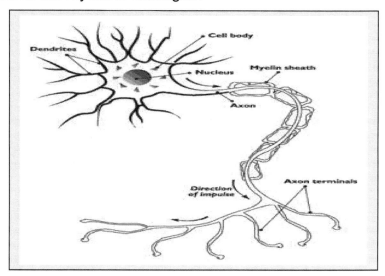

Fats = Hormones and little hormones (eicosanoids)

Cholesterol, a type of waxy fat, is the core molecule from which many hormones are manufactured. For instance, your body takes fat, adds a few attachments and produces DHEA, estrogen, progesterone and cortisol - hormones necessary for a healthy life.

Eicosanoids are hormone-like molecules that relay messages throughout the body triggering such diverse things as blood clotting and inflammation. They are also made from fat. Fats are in a constant, dynamic flux – sometimes functioning as material for cell membranes and at other times becoming eicosanoid messengers moving between cells. It's as if a brick from the foundation of a house were also able to carry messages to the neighbors. We have an amazingly dynamic body.

Fats = Padding and cushioning

Fat also pads joints and cushions the body from trauma. Most of this padding should, however, be invisible – surrounding the eyes, in joint spaces and lightly wrapped around organs and not hanging off the body.

Conclusion: Fat for life

You may or may not care about the details of fat and technical words. What is important is that fats matter.

Quality fats make an everyday difference in your health. You don't have to understand the chemistry to realize that

Regularly eating a Variety of Whole Organic oils can mean the difference between living well and suffering needlessly

---

.

Review

Fats, fatty acids and fat heads

There are thousands of different fats. They can be generally categorized as:

- Saturated
- Unsaturated
  - Monounsaturated
  - Polyunsaturated

Consistency/melting points of fats:

	Room Temperature	Refrigerated
Saturated Fats	Solid	Solid
Monunsaturated	Liquid	Semi-solid
Polyunsaturated	Liquid	Liquid

Basic Fatty Acids

The basic structure of fatty acids looks like this:

Methyl Group	Carbon Chain	Carboxyl Group
H_3C	CH_2	-COOH
Omega end	Variable length	

<------------- Fatty -------------><---- Acid ---->

There are many fatty acids. Their names and properties change depending on the number of carbon atoms. The fatty acid shown here is know as butyric acid. It is commonly found in butter. Is it saturated? Yes. Each carbon (C) has hydrogen (H) attached. The carbon parking spaces are filled with hydrogen cars preventing oxygen cars from parking. Its chemical formula is $C_4H_8O_2$.

Sometimes skeletal representations are used to visualize molecules. Butyric acid's is:

Saturated Fatty Acids

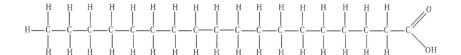

Stearic Acid is found in beef and lamb. Note that each C (carbon) has H (hydrogen) molecules attached making this a **saturated fat**. The hydrogen prevents oxygen from attaching to the carbon. This makes the molecule more stable and less susceptible to oxygenation which causes rancidity.

Other saturated fats are found in palm and coconut oil. Note that saturation is **not the same as cholesterol**. Palm and coconut oils are saturated, but contain no cholesterol.

Cholesterol

Cholesterol: In addition to the fatty acid chain (CH2-CH2) it contains ring structures that are used as the foundation of sterol molecules in the formation of **hormones** and other useful compounds. Cholesterol is so important for health, that it is not dependent on diet, but is formed in the liver.

Unsaturated Fatty Acids

1. **Monounsaturated fats**
2. **Polyunsaturated fats**

1. Monounsaturated Fats

Mono = one unsaturated site.

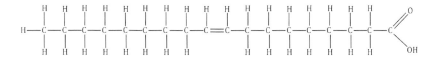

Oleic Acid: Commonly found in olive oil.

The Omega end (CH3) is followed by 17 carbons.

Oleic Acid is an 18 carbon molecule. Note at the 9th carbon there is a double bond (=). This makes oleic acid an omega-9 fatty acid. Numbering always starts from the left (the omega position). Double bonds open up space for oxygen to move in and attach to carbon atoms. This makes monounsaturated fats less stable than saturated fats, but more stable than polyunsaturated fats.

2. Polyunsaturated Fats Acids (PUFA)

Poly = many unsaturated sites

Two major types:

A. Omega-6 fatty acids
B. Omega-3 fatty acids

A. **Omega-6 Oils**

Found primarily in vegetables.

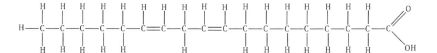

Linoleic Acid (LA):

An 18 carbon fatty acid with the first double bond (=) at the 6th carbon making it an omega-6 fatty acid. It has two double bonds.

Linoleic Acid (LA) converts to **pro-inflammatory** molecules:

- Prostaglandin E-2 (PGE-2)
- Thromboxane -2 (TXA-2)
- Leukotienes

B. **Omega-3 Oils**

Found primarily in fish, organic vegetables, grass-fed meat, chicken and dairy products.

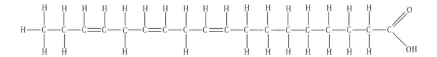

Alpha-linolenic Acid (ALA):

An 18 carbon fatty acid with the first double bond (=) at the 3rd carbon making it an omega-3 fatty acid. It has 3 double bonds. Alpha-linolenic Acid (ALA) is modified to form **EPA and DHA.**

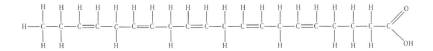

Eicosapentaenoic Acid (EPA)

An 18 carbon molecule with the first double bond at the 3rd carbon making it an omega-3 fatty acid. Note there are 5 double bonds making EPA more susceptible to oxygen attack.

EPA converts to **anti-inflammatory:**
- Prostaglandin-2 series (PGE-3)
- Thromboxane -3 (TXA-3)

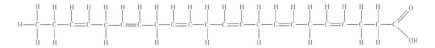

Docosahexaenoic Acid (DHA)

A 22 carbon molecule with the first double bond at the 3rd position making this also an omega-3 fatty acid. Note there are 5 double bonds to be attacked by oxygen.

- **DHA** is high in the brain and nervous system. We are all fat heads!
- **EPA and DHA**, because they are highly unsaturated, are the most vulnerable to oxidation.

Triglycerides

Another major fat is the group known as triglycerides. They come in many configurations and are important as an energy source (all tissues except the brain utilize triglycerides as energy), energy storage (also known as fat accumulation), padding, as a source of free fatty acids which can be utilized for numerous purposes, and as a storage for excess glucose intake. (Excess sugar converts into triglycerides, thus reducing sugar's damage to tissues. Diabetics will often see triglyceride levels increase along with their glucose levels.)

$$CH_2—OOC—R$$
$$|$$
$$CH—OOC—R'$$
$$|$$
$$CH_2—OOC—R''$$

| Glycerol Foundation | Fatty acid chains R = variable carbon chain. |

Linoleic Acid (LA) in food

Safflower Oil	78%	Sesame Oil	45%
Grape Seed Oil	73%	Rice Bran Oil	39%
Poppy Seed Oil	70%	Pistachio Oil	32.7%
Sunflower Oil	68%	Canola Oil	21%
Hemp Oil	60%	Egg Yolk	16%
Corn Oil	59%	Linseed oil	15%
Wheat Germ Oil	55%	Lard	10%
Cottonseed Oil	54%	Olive Oil	10%
Soybean Oil	51%	Palm Oil	10%
Walnut Oil	51%	Cocoa Butter	3%
Peanut Oil	48%	Macadamia	2%

Alpha-linolenic Acid (ALA) content of foods

Common name	Alternate name	Linnaean name	% ALA
Chia	chia sage	*Salvia hispanica*	64%
Kiwifruit seeds	gooseberry	*Actinidia chinensis*	62%
Perilla	shiso	*Perilla frutescens*	58%
Flax	linseed	*Linum usitatissimum*	55%
Lingonberry	cowberry	*Vaccinium vitis-idaea*	49%
Purslane	portulaca	*Portulaca oleracea*	35%
Sea Buckthorn	seaberry	*Hippophae rhamnoides L.*	32%
Hemp	cannabis	*Cannabis sativa*	20%
Rapeseed	canola	*Brassica napus*	10%
Soybean	soya	*Glycine max*	8%

Omega- 6 & omega-3 fatty acids in foods:

Name of the oil	Omega-6 fatty acids %	Omega-3 fatty acids %
Canola oil	22	10
Flaxseed oil	17	55
Safflower	76	Trace
Sunflower	71	1
Corn oil	57	1
Olive oil	9	1
Soybean oil	54	8
Coconut oil	2	0
Peanut oil	33	Trace

Most diets contain larger amounts of omega-6 oils than omega-3, creating an imbalance that leads to higher incidence of inflammation. Coconut oil is mostly saturated, containing little unsaturated oil, but no cholesterol.

Chapter 10

Fats 202 - More food for fat thought

History of Fat

In light of the rapid changes in fat consumption over the past 50 to 100 years, I think it's useful to look at the history of fat in case you missed Fat Class at school or have become dumbfounded by the media over this sticky issue.

Really Old Fat

Hunter-gatherers sharpened stone axes and used them for cracking nuts and killing fish as well as killing and butchering large mammals. They are believed to have smashed bones open to eat the fatty marrow. Toward the end of the Paleolithic period, with better tool-making and scarcer large animals, people increasingly caught fish on bone fish-hooks, collected shellfish and trapped and ate smaller mammals such as rabbits, birds and reptiles including snakes, crocodiles and turtles. Researchers believe the evolution of humans benefited from the higher levels of EPA oils in these foods. And, remember, they were only eating ORGANIC foods.

Historically, cradles of civilization tended to occur in areas with high availability of omega-3 oils. It is believed that this intake contributed to advances in brain function. The brain and nervous system contain high levels of omega-3 oil. Remember from Fats 101 that omega-3 EFAs are more liquid than saturated fats. This liquid nature allows for easier and faster nerve communications.

More recent fats

Early Romans and Greeks ate a high fat diet, but were generally lean and valued fitness highly. Their fats were primarily from nuts, olives, avocados and fish – high in monounsaturated and omega-3 polyunsaturated oils.

Geographical Fat

Populations such as Eskimos and other native peoples of the far north and south traditionally ate diets very high in fats. These were mostly the "good" omega-3 oils from fish.

As a rule, these populations were lean and fit although they consumed a much higher intake of fats than even the most fast-food addicted modern American. The rate of heart attack of Greenland Eskimos was only 10 percent that of U.S. adults. Obesity, diabetes, arthritis and other chronic disease rates were insignificant.

Unfortunately, these high-fat consuming populations have increasingly introduced highly-processed, high-sugar Western foods into their diets. While Western societies introduced these foods over hundreds of years, these people did it in one generation. As a result, they suffer four times the national average of diabetes, and are experiencing alarming increases in obesity and heart disease. They've gone from whale blubber to Twinkies in a generation and are suffering from it.

Granddad's bacon and eggs

What about the often-told story of the grandparent that lived to be 90 and ate bacon and drank whole milk every day?

Of course it's impossible to extract much useful information from anecdotal stories like these, but one thing is for certain - and perhaps critical. You do not eat the same quality or types of fats as your great-grandparents. What they ate was predominantly organic. Before large-scale factory farming, animals and plants were healthier and richer in nutrients. Your grandparents or great-grandparents if you're under 50) ate a radically different composition of oils – more omega-3s and fewer polyunsaturated fats. Yes, it is modern chemistry that has made corn, soy and other polyunsaturated oils readily available for mass consumption.

A number of researchers are looking into the health consequences of the change in oil consumption that has happened in the last 100 years. During this time, vegetable oil use has gone from being practically nonexistent to spreading around the globe. I've seen advertisements for corn oil in Indonesia - a very un-traditional plant and oil source for that part of the world. Customarily Indonesians and other tropical Asian populations ate saturated fat from coconut and omega-3 oils from seafood. Now they eat imported polyunsaturated oils and their health is in decline. I couldn't find coconut oil in grocery stores in Thailand!

> *"Your grandparents and great-grandparents ate a radically different composition of oils – more omega-3s and fewer polyunsaturated fats."*

Vegetable oils, except for olive, flax, nuts and seeds, are relatively difficult to extract. Corn and most vegetable seeds require modern machinery and chemicals to give up their oils. Until recently humans did not eat these oils except as part of the whole food. Yes, the Chinese have extracted soy oil for thousands of years, but not for use as a food; it was used as a fuel for heat and light.

Over the past couple of hundred years, omega-6 oil intake from corn, soy and other plants has gone up, while omega-3 intake plummeted. Our ancestors consumed omega-3 oils as fish, but also in grass-fed animals and organic vegetables.

Researchers believe this rise in omega-6 oil usage and lowered omega-3 intake is contributing to a number of medical problems including cancer and depression.

Fat consumption statistics

Since 1910, the average U.S. vegetable-oil consumption increased from 21 to 70 grams per day, while consumption of animal fat decreased slightly, from 104 to 99 grams/day. Consumption of beef and poultry increased while pork consumption decreased. The fat content of poultry also increased – due to factory farming.

Overall, fat intake has remained essentially constant, while the use of some meats has diminished.

Butter consumption declined to 1/5 of its 1910 level, while the use of margarine has increased. Margarine is made from polyunsaturated oils. Lard (the fat from animals) consumption fell by about one-fifth of its former level. Use of vegetable shortenings almost doubled. Consumption of edible beef fat rose by two and a half times because factory beef contains more fat than grass-fed. The intake of vegetable salad and cooking oils has increased by about 12 times.

Consumption of whole milk is less than one-half of its 1910 level. Cream intake is less than one-third the 1910 level. Cheese intake tripled. Ice cream and frozen desserts increased five times and low-fat milk consumption increased by a factor of three.

Cholesterol intake has remained essentially constant during the last 70 years as saturated fat increased 16 percent. Make note of two trends: (a) Decreased lard use in cooking, but increased fat in meat created an overall increase of saturated fat and (b) Organic and grass-fed animal consumption (which is higher in omega-3 oils) declined, while non-organic factory meat high in saturated fat rose.

Consumption of oleic acid (mainly as olive oil) is up 55 percent. Linoleic acid, from vegetable oil, is up 170 percent.

All of these changes in fat consumption increased the amount of polyunsaturated omega-6 oils and decreased the percentage of fish and organic food intake of omega-3 oils. This has created a serious imbalance. It is estimated that omega-3 oil intake has decreased to one sixth of its 1850 level.

Intake of unrefined oils rich in nutrients became rare in the past 100 years. The only remaining healthy oil used in significant levels is extra-virgin olive oil. (Although a 2007 article in *The New Yorker* revealed large-scale fraud in the olive industry; soy and other cheaper oils are sometimes used to extend olive oil or are outright substituted for olive oil.)

Organic meat and dairy intake has declined along with small farming, thus further reducing omega-3 intake and increasing saturated fat.

The good news is that there is an increasing consumption of organic products in the past 20 years. So, a small percentage of the population is increasing their omega-3 levels, while the vast majority are decreasing it.

What to make of all these figures? **Cholesterol intake cannot be the primary cause of cardiovascular disease because consumption has remained about the same in the last 100 years, while cardiovascular disease (CVD) has skyrocketed.** More likely culprits in the rise of CVD are trans-fatty acids, altered vegetable fats, high omega-6 to omega-3 ratios (increasing inflammation), and deficiencies of minerals and vitamins. Modern researchers are increasingly pointing a finger at these as the cause of higher levels of cardiovascular and cancer deaths.

How can butter be blamed when its consumption has

gone down? In 1900, when people ate butter, CVD accounted for one in seven deaths. In 1980, when butter was avoided, CVD accounted for one in two deaths. Since 1980, CVD deaths have declined to more than one in three. This improvement is not due to any change in fat consumption, but to better post-heart attack management and increased consumption of vitamins, especially vitamin C.

Essential Fatty Acid Imbalances

Health problems can result when the ratio of omega-6 to omega-3 EFAs becomes imbalanced.

It has been estimated that between 1909 and 1985 omega-6 intake increased from 1kg/year to 12 kg/yr due to increased vegetable oil consumption. At the same time, omega-3 oil consumption went down. The ratio of omega-6 to omega-3 has increased from 4:1 to 25:1 (so 25 times more omega-6 than omega-3). Some researchers believe that early human consumption of omega-6 and omega-3 oils was 1:1, or equal, and that current levels may be as high as 30:1. This historic high omega-3 oil consumption coincided with the period of rapid brain development.

Whatever the exact ratio, we know that it is much different than it was even as little as 100 years ago. This change in fat intake is another example of the dramatic

> *"This change in fat intake is another example of the dramatic changes our bodies have been subjected to in a relatively short period of time."*

changes our bodies have been subjected to in a relatively short period of time.

Remember from the chapters on fats, omega-6 oils promote clotting, inflammation and muscle spasms, while omega-3 oils decrease clotting, inflammation and spasm (not just in your leg muscle, but also in your blood vessels). You can see then why the current imbalance in fat intake is correlated with an increased tendency to inflammation, more rigid cell membranes (impaired cellular communication), higher risk for cancer, greater post-menopausal bone loss, auto-immune disease, diabetes and cardiovascular disease.

Do you have an EFA imbalance?

Imbalances in EFAs are extremely common in the U.S. and are responsible for a number of chronic health conditions.

How do you know if you're low? Laboratory tests are available. Signs and symptoms of an EFA deficiency or imbalance include such things as dry skin, dry hair, eczema, depression and learning problems. If you have a chronic inflammatory condition such as heart and vascular disease, arthritis, asthma, dermatitis, or irritable bowel disease – yes, these are all inflammatory diseases - you should talk to your naturopath about your oil intake and digestion.

But I thought vegetable oil was good for me!

I know, you've been told to use vegetable oils, but think about what your ancestors consumed. They could not easily extract oil from corn and soy. This requires machinery and chemicals. Your ancestors' diet was high in monounsaturated fats from olives, nuts and seeds and omega-3 oils from fish, flax, walnut, hemp, borage and green leafy vegetables. Grass-fed meat and dairy also contain significant amounts of omega-3 oil (unlike grain-fed products).

Your genetic material and chemical balances "grew up" relying on omega-3 oils (and a high intake of antioxidants to keep them from going rancid).

Some individuals exhibit biochemical individuality in the way they process EFAs. Their reduced level of an important enzyme (delta-6 desaturase) reduces the production of important prostaglandins. These people are even more reliant on the intake of fish and organic meats as a source of EFAs and don't do as well with flax and other vegetable sources.

What affects omega-3 levels?

You must first eat these good oils. Secondly, you must digest them. Micronutrient deficiencies (B3, B6, Biotin, C, zinc, magnesium, and chromium) can alter balances of EFAs.

Excessive blood glucose also upsets EPA balance in favor of the pro-inflammatory omega-6, arachidonic acid pathway. A high carbohydrate/low protein/low fiber diet is not just a recipe for adult-onset diabetes; it increases inflammation and clotting, leading to a greater likelihood of stroke.

Fresh wild fish (not farm raised) is the best source of omega-3 oils. While EFA capsules are often helpful, the bioavailability of these oils from fish may be greater. One researcher, Claudio Galli, PhD, Professor at the Institute of Pharmacological Sciences, University of Milan, reports that plasma DHA levels following the consumption of 308 mg DHA from smoked salmon were double those obtained from 1680 mg provided in capsules. On the other hand, good-quality fish oils have removed the mercury and other contaminants that may be found in fish.

What do I do to raise my omega-3 levels?

Consuming whole foods, by promoting monounsaturated and omega-3 oil intake from fish and organic foods, is the best way to overcome the ill effects of EFA imbalances.

Fat be bad?

As I've explained, fats are necessary to life and health. But like most anything else, fats can be bad for you if not used in a healthy way. The main problems with fat have to do with excess intake, poor quality, and hydrogenation.

Excess Intake

Quality is more important than quantity, but there are people who eat too many fats. It is more common for the person who is eating bad fats to consume excessive amounts. Eating good quality fats is nutritionally more satisfying and filling. In other words, some people eat too much fat because they're starved for good fat. Their body keeps crying out for good-quality EFAs.

How much fat?

There is considerable debate of this question. Current consumption in the American diet is about 35 percent of total calories. The American Cancer Society and the American Heart Association recommend a diet of less than 30 percent of calories derived from fat.

Thirty to 35 percent is probably less than what Paleolithic peoples consumed and is certainly less than Eskimos traditionally ate. In general, the colder the climate, the more fat was included in the diet. Most of the evidence shows that these high-fat diets of traditional foods were not harmful. These people generally had low rates of heart disease, cancer and diabetes until they converted to Western diets.

Current Mediterranean diets from Italy, Greece and Crete contain about 30 percent fat. These people have a low incidence of heart and blood vessel disease. Their intake of omega-3 oils (from fish, vegetables, nuts, flax) is higher than their intake of vegetable oils (from corn, soy, safflower, and cottonseed) and they consume less hydrogenated oils. In other words, while the quantity is relatively high, the quality is excellent.

Your perfect fat level

Calculating the "perfect" level of fat intake for yourself is, in most cases, unnecessary. If you follow the Three Wisdoms, you will probably consume somewhere in the range of 25 to 35 percent fats. More importantly, all your fats will be of good quality, in the correct ratios and un-hydrogenated. A whole-food, organic diet makes it difficult to over-consume fats.

Even if you only followed one aspect of the Three Wisdoms - avoiding processed foods - you will have eliminated a large portion of the problem that affects most Western peoples: hidden, poor-quality fats.

It is common for my patients on the **Nutrition-1-2-3** program to lose their craving for fatty foods. Once they supply their cells with high-quality lipids, their body's inner wisdom takes over.

Calculating your fat intake

One advantage of following the Three Wisdoms is that much of the hassle of issues like counting calories and figuring fat intake is taken care of. When you're Regularly eating a Variety of Whole foods, portion size, calories and fats are usually consumed at healthy levels. On the other hand, some people find it helpful to track their fat intake for a while.

Figuring the right ratio of fat is slightly more difficult than keeping track of carbs and protein because fats contain more calories per weight. Fat has nine calories per gram while protein and starch each have four. In other words, protein and starch have the same number of calories per gram, while fat has over twice as many calories per gram. For orientation, there are 28 grams in an ounce and eight ounces in a cup.

Remember, food labels (see Nibbles at end of book) list ingredients by grams, not by percentage of calories. You need to make the simple calculation changing grams to percentages. Since proteins and carbs have the same number of calories per gram, then the grams and percentages are the same. That is, 40 grams of carbs and 20 grams of protein equals a 40/20 ratio. But, for figuring percentages of calories from fat, you multiply the grams of fat by two to achieve a comparison. That's because there are twice as many calories per gram of fat.

For example, a food label might list a portion size as 40 grams of carbs, 30 grams of protein and 15 grams of fat. The calorie percentages are then 40/30/30 because you've multiplied fat's 15 grams by 2 to come up with 30. A more complicated calculation, but one you can do in your head, is 30 grams of carbs, 10 grams of protein and 20 grams of fat. Your percentage of calories would then be 30/10/40 (carbs/protein/fat). In this example, the protein is too low and the fat is too high if your goal is a 40/30/30 ratio. This is typical of many packaged foods and one reason why I suggest you use them sparingly.

General guidelines for estimating protein, fat and carb content of foods:

- Vegetables and fruits (except avocados): Consider them 100% starch and sugars.
- Beans and grains: A combination of carbohydrates and protein with very little fat.
- Nuts and seeds: Fat, protein, with a small amount of carbohydrates. (Brazil nuts have lots of fat. Almonds are highest in protein. Hazel nuts have more carbohydrates.)
- Dairy products: Protein, fat (unless it was removed) and carbs. (Milk has more carbohydrates while cottage cheese has more protein.)
- Meat, chicken, fish, eggs: Primarily protein. Fat depends on how it was raised and the cut. Few carbohydrates.

Let's try one more example: Ten grams of carbs, 30 grams of protein and 5 grams of fat. What are the calorie percentages? Answer: 10/30/10. You might see these numbers on a truly high-protein bar, but it's rare.

I know that if you're not used to these numbers it can

be a bit confusing at first. After a week or two this will all become second nature. And you don't need to be precise in your calculations. Rounding off numbers is fair in nutrition.

What about calculating fat percentage of foods with no labels? The only way to do that is to know the percentage breakdown of each food. For this you need a specialized book that lists foods with their percentages of carbs, proteins, and fats. I recommend you spend your time with your family and friends, not making exact calculations.

Ballpark estimations of percentages can be made by knowing generally how much fat is in food.

Again, food categories vary widely in their composition. That is one reason eating a Variety of food is so important.

Very-low-fat diets

Several researches including Dean Ornish, MD, have written books recommending extremely low-fat diets of 5 to 10 percent. Their results were favorable at reversing existing heart disease.

Five to 10 percent fat is less than what most researchers believe comprised traditional diets. This is also very difficult for most people to adhere to. The body needs fat and craves it.

An example of the difficulty of controlling fat intake comes from the Women's Health Initiative, a study of nearly 49,000 women randomly assigned to follow a low-fat diet or not. Despite extensive and expensive counseling, 69 percent of those assigned to a low-fat diet were not able to cut their fats to 20 percent. In other words only 31 percent kept to the low-fat diet. You could interpret this as a lack of will power. My feeling is that our bodies require more than 20 percent fat and will compel us to eat it no matter what inducements researchers offer.

There are also other factors besides a specific amount of fat that contribute to the success of the low-fat diet. The true Ornish diet is not only low in fat, but high in complex carbohydrates and fiber while low in refined carbohydrates. This definitely contributes to the success of this diet in countering heart disease. Just how much of the benefit comes from low fat and how much from other dietary factors such as high fiber and vegetable nutrients is uncertain. These factors are very difficult to control for in real-world scientific studies.

Another issue that makes the Ornish diet difficult to evaluate is that his subjects weren't just eating a low-fat diet; they were eating a low **bad-fat** diet. The benefit of the low-fat diet may have more to do with reducing poor quality fats than the overall quantity. By reducing overall fat in a typical American non-organic diet, you reduce your intake of pesticides, herbicides, hormones, antibiotics, hydrogenation, and rancidity. The Standard American Diet (SAD) is high in bad fats.

It's interesting to note that another population group that enjoys relatively good health is the Japanese. They eat far less fat than the classic Mediterranean diet. A paradox: two healthy groups that consume radically different levels of fat. The common denominators: Seafood and good-quality fats.

Except for a person with known heart disease dieting under a physician's supervision, I would not suggest a very low-fat diet. The healthy choice and one easier to maintain would be to trade in all your bad fats for good ones by following the Third Wisdom – Whole Foods: fresh, unprocessed and organic.

The problem with dietary guidelines

While the American Dietetic Association (ADA) and American Heart Associations (AHA) may be correct in recommending you reduce your fats, I believe their suggested methods are wrong. Rather than pick on meat and dairy consumption, they should tell people to:

- Only eat fat from organically-raised plants and animals. These fats contain lower saturated and higher polyunsaturated fats and don't have the various poisons associated with non-organic – pesticides, hormones, and antibiotics.

- Avoid hydrogenated fat. If people followed this advice, they would reduce their fat intake, eliminate a toxic form of fat and greatly reduce junk food from their diet. Most processed foods contain hydrogenated fat, as well as too much fat and sugar overall.

- Eat more omega-3 rich foods such as fish and organic meat, dairy and eggs.

By concentrating on the quality of fat intake, the ADA and AHA could do much more for people's health. Excess weight, heart disease, diabetes, cancer, and multiple other problems are better controlled with whole, fresh, organic foods.

Hydrogenation and trans-fatty acids

Hydrogenation is a process by which vegetable oils that are liquid at room temperature are hardened by the addition of hydrogen atoms to binding sites. Again, picture the oil as a parking garage and the carbon atoms as parking spaces. By adding more hydrogen "cars" the spaces fill up and the liquid oil becomes hard. You are familiar with this in your kitchen as the corn or soy oil that has been hardened into a butter-like solidness called margarine.

Hydrogenated oils are also found in many processed foods such as chips, French fries, ice cream, donuts, candy, cookies, salad dressing and peanut butter. Reading food labels (see Nibbles at end of book), if you buy foods with labels, is the best way to find if a food contains hydrogenated oil. If it has hydrogenated oil then it has trans-fatty acids.

During hydrogenation a portion of the polyunsaturated fatty acids (PUFAs) are converted to trans-fatty acids. Trans-fatty acids are corrupted fats with a backward shape. They are not found in natural foods. Hydrogenated foods are particularly high in trans-fatty acids. Hydrogenated oils supply 80 percent of the trans-fatty acids found in the typical American diet.

Hydrogenated oils were first introduced to the public in 1911. Since then, the total average intake of trans-fatty acids from hydrogenated oils has risen from zero to close to 10 percent or between 10 and 15 grams (0.5 ounces) per person per day.

The problem with these oils is that they are not natural to the body. They become twisted into unnatural shapes. Cells don't recognize them as something they've seen before. Hydrogenated fats cross into the placenta, the brain, liver, heart and cell membranes. They contain no nutritional value, only calories and risk of disease.

Intakes of hydrogenated and trans-fatty acids are associated with increased cholesterol levels, risk of heart attack and cancer. The long-term health effects of these industrial byproducts have not been studied and are unknown. Consumers are the guinea pigs.

> According to Dr. Ralph Holman, a Mayo Clinic researcher, "Large scale hydrogenation of vegetable oils reduces omega-3 and omega-6 fatty acids and replaces them with saturated and trans-fatty acids that interfere with the omega-3 and omega-6 metabolism, inducing significant partial deficiencies of essential fatty acids."

Pregnant women who consume trans-fatty acids have babies with more trans and less DHA, the fatty acid that plays a critical role in brain, sight and nerve development, according to a 2001 report in the *Journal of Clinical Nutrition*.

Hydrogenated oils compete with essential fatty acids for uptake into all cells of the body. In some cases this can cause a deficiency of the essential oil for building cells. These oils interfere with cell membrane flexibility, fluid dynamics, and the production of omega-3 oils.

Unlike the SAD diet, the Three Wisdoms diet contains no hydrogenated oils.

By the way, the research on the evils of trans-fats is not new. I studied it 30 years ago. If you see an MD for high cholesterol, heart disease, or cancer, ask why he or she didn't warn you about these before they recently became newspaper headlines.

How antioxidants save your life every day

Free Radicals

There is a gang of thugs that hang out in your body. They're called free radicals and they can do a lot of damage, if you let them.

Free radicals are molecules or ions, usually containing oxygen, that only have a single electron instead of the usual two. (Remember electrons? They "spin" around the nucleus of a nucleus.) Free radicals do damage by stealing electrons from other molecules. Free radicals also like to multiply rapidly, creating whole gangs of bad-dude molecules.

Polyunsaturated fatty acids are particular targets of free radical damage. Remember, they contain many parking sites for oxygen free radicals to park. Outside the body, vegetable oils that are exposed to oxygen are prone to oxidative destruction. Heating the oil increases the problem.

Free radicals attack enzymes, DNA and cell membranes. Many health conditions have been associated with their damage: arthritis, Alzheimer's disease, high blood pressure, cancer, hardening of the arteries, lung disease, aging, senility and Parkinson's disease, to name a few.

Your load of free radicals is also increased by exposure to ultraviolet light, X-rays, radon and other forms of ionizing radiation. Ozone and nitrogen oxide are also converted into free radicals. These damaging little guys are so abundant that it is estimated that they initiate 10,000 attacks on your DNA every day. Fortunately DNA repair proteins usually repair this damage.

> *"Polyunsaturated fatty acids are particular targets of free-radical damage."*

Free radicals are actually a normal part of body chemistry. Your cells make them while using oxygen to produce energy. For instance, the liver produces free radicals as a byproduct during detoxification of pollutants and toxic chemicals.

Antioxidants

The gang of free radicals is not unopposed. Antioxidants are free radical scavengers. They block the oxidation of free-radicals and their subsequent damage. Tough antioxidants include vitamins E and C. There are also enzymes that prevent free radical attack, including catalase, superoxide dismutase and glutathione peroxidase.

Some of the trace minerals also act as antioxidants. Zinc, copper, manganese and selenium are important co-factors in the antioxidant process. Plant micronutrients called carotenoids, including the well-known beta-carotene, as well as hundreds of other carotenoids, also act as antioxidants.

Vegetables and fruits, because of their abundance of

carotenoids, vitamins and minerals, are great sources of antioxidants. This is why they are so effective in preventing heart disease and cancer as well as other health problems. Organic, fresh vegetables and fruits are the best way of insuring that you're consuming enough antioxidants.

Whole foods keep the free radical thugs in check.

Fat summary

I hope I've made the point that fats, in the form of good fats, are vital for your health. You may need to reduce your overall fat intake, but more importantly you need to eliminate bad fats and increase your consumption of high-quality fats, especially the omega-3 family. Antioxidants protect oils from the damaging effects of heat and oxygen. The Three Wisdoms program is the optimal eating program for keeping your fats - and yourself - healthy.

Chapter 11

Micronutrients 101 -

Good things in small packages

Now that we've discussed the big nutrients (macronutrients) - carbohydrates, proteins and fats – let's catch up on the small, but vitally important, micronutrients.

Vitamins: vital for life

Vitamins are nutrients that are essential for life. They are also "organic." Organic in this case refers to the chemistry definition meaning they contain the element carbon. Most of us are more familiar with the other definition of organic, meaning raised naturally without pesticides, herbicides, and genetically-modified organisms.

Vitamins are necessary for three general functions of the body:

- **Growth**
- **Protection**
- **Energy regulation**.

There are 13 commonly recognized vitamins and they are classified as fat soluble or water soluble, meaning they either dissolve in fat or in water.

Fat soluble vitamins

Vitamins A, D, E and K.

Water Soluble vitamins

Vitamins B (there are eight) and C.

Vitamins: They must come from food

A basic but often misunderstood rule of nature is that the body cannot synthesize enough vitamins to sustain life. Generally, they must come in through the diet. There are a couple of exceptions to this. Vitamin D can be manufactured by the skin if it is exposed to sufficient sunlight. Biotin and pantothenic acid (two B vitamins) and vitamin K can be synthesized in the intestines by healthy bacteria.

Unfortunately, most modern foods, grown with artificial fertilizer and later processed, are deficient in vitamins. This is well documented by the US Department of Agriculture (USDA) and other research groups. For some inexplicable reason, the medical industry refuses to accept the correlation between vitamin deficiencies and disease.

Vitamin History

Vitamin A was the first vitamin discovered. That was in 1912. Before qualifying as a vitamin, it is necessary to prove that the compound must be obtained from the diet to sustain life.

Vitamin Function

It is not necessary for you to know what each vitamin does in the body. For one thing, the list is too long. For instance, while vitamin D is mainly thought of as an aid to bone growth and strength, it also can act as a mood elevator, immune system support, and hormone regulator. We also know it helps protect us from certain types of cancer. There is no end to the list of good things vitamins do for us.

Basically, all you need to know is that vitamins are necessary for health and life. You might say that carbohydrates, proteins and fats are the building blocks and vitamins make them work.

Minerals: More life support

Minerals are elements that are inorganic (non-carbon containing). You've probably seen a periodic chart of the elements at some point in your schooling. This chart lists all the minerals necessary for life, plus some extras. Calcium, magnesium, zinc, copper, manganese, chromium, potassium, selenium, cobalt, iron, sodium, iodine, sulfur, phosphorus, chloride, fluoride, and molybdenum are the minerals necessary for life. Uranium is not necessary.

Minerals, like vitamins, must be taken in through the diet and are necessary for health and life. And like vitamins, each performs many functions.

Mineral Functions – a few examples

Building blocks

Calcium and magnesium for bones.

Activating enzymes

Potassium for transmission of nerve impulses and muscle contractions.

Control of body processes

Chloride for balancing acid and alkaline levels. Sodium for maintaining blood volume.

Mineral Sources

Minerals come from the soil and are taken up by plants. If the soil is deficient, as it is in most of the U.S., then the plant will be deficient. This is where artificial fertilizers go wrong. They are not a balance of all the minerals we need to be healthy. Composting, as practiced by organic farmers, provides the full spectrum of minerals.

Minerals and Health

Minerals are necessary for health and life. Sadly, the food and beverage industries largely ignore this fact. Quantity - the size of the plant – matters more than the quality of nutrients in the plant. While it is well-documented by the USDA and other researchers, the declining quality of our foods and its impact on our health is almost totally ignored by the medical community.

Other nutrients

Countless other nutrients that do not qualify as vitamins and minerals have been discovered. There are probably more that have yet to be discovered. Our knowledge of the role of micronutrients in life and health is very limited.

For instance, there are over 500 carotenoids, the family of nutrients of which beta-carotene is a member. They account for the color or pigmentation in foods, but are also crucial as antioxidants and immune enhancers. While not classified as vitamins, they protect us from cancer, heart disease and other conditions.

Micronutrients in your life

Your health is dependent on vitamins, minerals and other micronutrients. Your hunter-gather ancestors ate an abundant variety of these nutrients. Modern foods are increasingly deficient in them and this deficiency predisposes you to illness.

Although needed in small amounts, micronutrients play a big role in health.

Chapter 12

Water -

The fourth food group

Water doesn't appear on most food charts or pyramids, but it is critical to life. You could argue that it's more important than food because you can live without food for weeks, but only a few days without water.

Water was the main drink of hunter-gatherers and only fell into disfavor as humans started living in unsanitary towns that poisoned their water supplies. Then beer and wine became popular. Alcohol helped build the pyramids and much of civilization. Today, juices, soda pop and coffee fuel the day.

Alarmingly, in the United States, more soda is consumed than water. The average yearly intake of soda is 40 gallons — a frightening experiment in ingesting fructose, FD&C colors and artificial sweeteners.

Researchers commonly find mild to moderate dehydration in average people. Dehydration is not a benign condition. It reduces the efficiency of the cells to carry out their processes — chemical reactions slow down, nutrients stagnate, and waste removal is delayed. This translates into reduced body energy and brain impairment.

Most weight-loss diets recommend water as an

important tool for increasing metabolism. Research (*Journal of Clinical Endocrinology and Metabolism*, December 2003) shows that water intake increases the rate at which people burn calories. A little more than two cups of water a day increased metabolism by an amazing 30 percent. This metabolic boost takes place within 10 minutes of drinking water. Researchers estimated that by consuming 1.5 liters of water a day, the average person would burn an extra 17,400 calories, for a weight loss of approximately five pounds per year.

Sometimes people eat or drink a calorie beverage when they are not really hungry, only thirsty. For instance, a recent study found that kids who drank more than three glasses of milk a day are prone to obesity. It was suggested they would be better off drinking more water.

How much water?

As you might guess, not a lot of money has gone into water research – except when its "fortified" as a sports drink. Most experts tend to use the figure of eight glasses of water each day. Those who work or exercise heavily need even more. If you have a tendency toward constipation, kidney stones or gallstones, water may keep you out of the emergency room. Some doctors recommend one gallon a day. As the research above showed, 1.5 liters increased metabolism, so that seems like a reasonable goal.

If you have a concern about additional water making it necessary for you to urinate too often, gradually increase your water over several weeks. If urination disturbs your sleep, drink the majority of your water before 3 p.m.

Can't stand the taste? A good filter, changed regularly, does wonders. Some people find that a squeeze of pure lemon or a tablespoon of organic fruit juice turns on their thirst buds.

Water with meals?

Some lay authors advise not to drink fluids during a meal. They claim this will dilute digestive enzymes and reduce digestive function. I have never seen this supported in any research studies or mentioned in nutrition textbooks.

- Most animals drink water, when available, with their food.
- If you have trouble digesting foods, don't stop drinking water, have your digestive function evaluated.
- Obviously you don't want to drink large amounts of water with a meal, but sipping a glass is fine.

What about other drinks?

I suggest sticking with what humans drank traditionally — water. Other acceptable beverages are herbal teas, green teas and very diluted fruit juices. Full-strength fruit juices have too much sugar, not enough fiber, and high concentrations of pesticides, unless they're organic.

Coffee and caffeinated teas and sodas are diuretics; they stimulate the kidneys to lose water through urination. Think of them as anti-water. They increase your need for real water. A recent study sponsored by The Coca-Cola Company disputes this and claims Coke is a fine water substitute. However, this was a pilot study only lasting one day and it even demonstrated a decrease in potassium among caffeinated beverage drinkers. Despite the study's shortcomings and obvious bias, it was quoted favorably by the media and even nutrition "experts". This is just another obvious example of the power of advertising over facts.

If you like coffee, drink it the way you would any herb or condiment; in small doses, organic, and with food — not alone. My major concern about coffee is that some people use it as a source of energy. If your energy is not good, do something about the problem; don't cover it up with a stimulant.

Bottled or tap water?

Many bottled waters are no more pure than good tap water, although this obviously depends on where you live. If the bottle is a soft plastic container, the plastic is known to leach into the water and has been associated with hormonal disruption and cancer. The plastic also contributes to land fill waste or increased recycling burden.

In addition, every time you purchase bottled water, you're helping to privatize what has been a public resource. Analysts expect three companies will control 65 to 75 percent of what are now public waterworks in Europe and North America in the next 15 years.

Home water filtration systems do an excellent job of removing problem chemicals and contaminants and are less expensive, in the long run, than bottled water. Filters are also more environmentally friendly and save room in your recycling bin. Check with *Consumer Reports* (www.consumerreports.com) to find their current recommendation as these devices keep improving. Obviously, they're only as good as the filter, so change yours regularly.

Water, more precious than oil

The growing scarcity of clean water for drinking has lead many environmental experts to predict that nations will soon be competing for water as viciously as they now battle for oil. Modern non-organic farming practices have increased the poisoning of the water table and increase water loss through evaporation. It's a sad state of affairs that leaves us now viewing this natural resource as a commodity.

Water, it's the evolutionary drink with no superior. Value it, conserve it, and drink it.

Chapter 13

At the table –

Sitting down with carbs, protein, fats, and micronutrients

You've probably seen the recommendations on food charts and pyramids to eat five to seven vegetables and fruit, three to four starches, two to three proteins and one or two oils each day. Few people meet these suggestions. Our ancestors undoubtedly exceeded them.

I encourage people to eat five servings (1/2 cup = 1 serving) of fruits and vegetables throughout the day as a minimum. There is virtually no maximum. Eating this amount of vegetables would probably cure three-quarters of those suffering from excess weight, diabetes, heart disease and all other chronic health conditions. Besides the added nutrients, people eating lots of fresh produce are less likely to eat processed foods and sugar.

Starches in the form of whole grains and baked goods need only be eaten in small quantities except for those needing more calories because they're doing hard physical labor or exercise.

I suggest protein is eaten at each meal and snack. This stabilizes the blood sugar and insulin levels.

Fats generally take care of themselves as many foods

contain them. Again, think quality.

What your plate should look like

When all is said and argued about food groups, between servings per day and percentages, what it boils down to is what you have on your plate when you sit down to eat. Hunter-gatherers would recognize a plate containing mostly green vegetables, some starchy vegetables and a protein portion such as fish or meat. If extra starch is needed for energy, a small amount of grain-based food or a potato will supply it. Fats would come from the fish or meat and also from nuts and seeds.

A word on portion size – the hand method

Portion sizes, especially in some restaurants, have gotten out of hand. It's no wonder that restaurants are now making their chairs bigger than they did thirty years ago.

Speaking of "out of hand", your hand comes in handy for measuring portion size. It's a good indicator of how much you should be eating.

A large protein portion is roughly the size of the palm of your hand. Starchy foods should be no bigger than your fist. Green leafy vegetables can be eaten in unlimited quantities since they have lots of nutritional value, but few calories.

Plate checklist

Here's a quick checklist to use when deciding what to put on your plate.

Total carbs

Does your meal contain a low, medium or high amount of carbs? My choice will depend on the amount of exercise I'm doing and when I last ate. Selecting a carb can be a little tricky because most foods are a mixture of protein, starch and fat. It's the ratios that are different. You want to know if the food is mostly starch (potatoes) or does it contain a decent amount of protein (millet, quinoa, or beans)?

It's not that I don't eat potatoes. My choice is based on how much protein and starch are in the other portions of this meal. Potatoes are fine if they are balanced with three ounces of chicken, fish (organic, naturally) or other concentrated protein. On the other hand, if the size of the protein is small or it is a protein that also contains starch (bean chili, for instance) then I'd be inclined to choose a carbohydrate with a higher percentage of protein.

A common example of a meal with possibly too much starch would be chips, tortillas, rice and beans in a Mexican restaurant, unless you're doing heavy exercise.

Type of carbs: Complex or simple?

The more complex the carbohydrates, the better. Many people don't realize that raisins and other dried fruits are high in sugars. You can't go wrong with vegetables. They're a great complex carb source. Complex carbs are also high in fiber.

Protein content

I find it easiest to have protein be the first thing I consider about any meal or snack. Once I know the amount of protein, I can look at the carbs. My target is in the range of 40 percent carbs, 30 percent protein and 30 percent fat. If you're reading labels, this calculation is easy because the protein, carbs and fats will be listed in grams.

For instance, if the carbohydrate portion of your meal is 40 grams, then the protein should be around 30 grams, or roughly a 4/3 ratio. If you're looking at a plate of home-cooked food – which I hope you're doing most of the time – then make your 40/30/30 calculation based on size using your hand as a measuring device.

Fats: Quality makes the difference

Interestingly, although the medical community and press have created a lot of confusion and hysteria over fats, they are usually the portion on your plate that you need to worry the least about. Whole, organic foods generally do not have too much fat and the quality is excellent. The only time you may need to scrutinize this portion of your meal is when you're eating in a restaurant or eating processed foods.

Micronutrients

Don't forget the little guys and girls

Is the food on your plate full of other nutrients? Vegetables such as carrots and broccoli are relatively high in carbohydrates when compared to chard and other green leafy vegetables, but are higher in carotenes, vitamins and minerals compared to crackers and breads. The choice would depend on creating the right balance of carbohydrates, proteins and other nutrients for you at that day's activity level. This again makes vegetables and fruits good carb sources, because they're also high in vitamins and minerals.

Your plate

Running through this sort of checklist takes a little time to put into practice at first but becomes second nature after a few weeks. It can make a huge difference in your energy levels and can help control your weight.

In the next section, we'll be applying the food groups to the Three Wisdoms.

> *"The more whole organic food you're eating, the less you have to worry about getting the "right" mix of nutrients because nature has done the balancing for you. Enjoy!"*

SECTION III

The Main Course

Chapter 14

From Confusion to Clarity - The Three Wisdoms

The heart of this book is about the wisdom of three concepts

- **Regularity**
- **Variety**
- **Wholeness**

First, we'll discuss how these Wisdoms are supported by history and science. Later chapters will expand their meaning in your kitchen, shopping cart and favorite restaurants. My goal is to make these concepts easy to understand and implement into your life.

Should food decisions be complicated?

It's a discouraging feeling to be a reasonably intelligent person, a high-school or even college graduate, able to hold down a job, raise children and even have a good handle on the difference between right and wrong, but still not know what to eat for breakfast. For many people, healthy eating no longer comes naturally. You probably know more about your car than you do your intake of protein. Food 101 is missing from basic education and Food 102 is absent from most medical visits.

Many people have given up worrying about diet, nutrition and anything resembling a food group. There are enough things pressing you for time. You need to pay bills. Your kids are asking for help with homework. Your spouse is in a bad/good mood. The lawn is past-due for a mowing. You haven't called your mother in a week. Your favorite TV show is on. Who has time to study nutrition, read labels, weigh portions, or be a careful shopper?

On the other hand, you haven't had any get-up-and-go in years. You'd rather not be watching TV, but don't have the energy to do anything else. Your kids are sick with ear aches and allergies all the time. Your spouse's blood pressure is high. After your gallbladder surgery, you were found to have high cholesterol and were put on medication. Even the family

> *"This is where most of my patients find themselves - not feeling well, but not knowing what to do about it."*

dog has been diagnosed with diabetes. (Pets, because they often have the same poor diets as humans, are increasingly developing arthritis, cancer, diabetes and the other diseases of modern human society.)

This is where most of my patients find themselves - not feeling well, but not knowing what to do about it. They may even have a sense that diet is part of their problem, but feel too confused by what they read to take action.

So, thinking that diet might help, you decide to do some research. You ask a friend about that new diet she just started. You read newspaper articles on the latest research on which foods are currently in or out of favor. You go to a bookstore and browse the sagging shelves of self-help diet books.

The problem: Confusion

Your friend Sally (not her real name) swears by her new kumquat diet. She's lost ten pounds! However, Sally has developed a chronic rash, her kids are exhibiting behavioral problems, and her husband has been "working late" every night since she proclaimed the kumquat diet edict. Yes, the weaknesses of fad diets soon reveal themselves.

The newspaper doesn't help. One day researchers say fat is bad. The following day it is reported that the Lipo people of New Oleo eat fat as a bedtime snack and live to be 200 years old.

On the internet bright colors and slick graphics encourage you to buy the one thing that will change your life. It must be great! Look at all the endorsements! (But no scientific support.)

At the bookstore you find the same confusing procession of opinions and proclamations. Some require a degree in biochemistry to understand, but none agree with the other. High protein? Low protein? Only vegetable protein? One book requires you to remodel your kitchen. A second forbids you from eating any animal with a tail. A degree in advanced calculus helps understand the measurements required for another program – and don't forget to carry your food scale everywhere.

What's a person to do? Do you give up? You can try to stop thinking about good health, but that would require you to give up reading, listening to the radio and watching TV. The media is full of funny, startling and scary tales of what to do and what not to do. Is this what they mean by "breaking news"?

You become increasingly frustrated and guilt-ridden. You should know more. You should do more. You feel you've lost control of a major portion of your life - eating - to glossy advertising and the precarious cravings of your appetite. But wait.

Good nutrition doesn't need to be complicated

No. It can actually be quite simple.

Gaining command over the media hype, the high-pressure sales and the "follow me" desperation of friends is easy if you have a solid foundation that guides you toward health.

Fortunately for you, the most reliable information about nutrition has not changed for tens of thousands of years. And this historic record of how to eat well has been verified by the best scientific research. This knowledge fills volumes, but is easily synthesized for your understanding.

As the next few chapters explain, planning, shopping and eating can be organized by three easy-to-remember concepts: (Yes, I'm saying it again, just in case you were dozing earlier.)

Regularity. Variety. Wholeness.

My goal is that by the end of this book you find Regularity, Variety and Wholeness easy to incorporate into your life and use them as touchstones for evaluating media reports, experts' claims and fad diets. Your health depends on you being well-armed against a world that thrives on confusion and misinformation.

Who gains from nutritional confusion? The food and medical industries.

Who loses? You.

Eating powerful, health-building meals isn't as complicated and confusing as you might think. I know; newspapers, magazines, radio, internet and TV aren't much help. In fact, they mostly add to the confusion.

You've been led to believe that good nutrition is an impossible dream, something no mortal can ever attain. I hope to change your mind. I believe that good nutrition can be synthesized into three words. These three words will guide you to better shopping, cooking, eating and health.

Back to Basics:

The Three Wisdoms - **Regularity, Variety and Wholeness** - are simple concepts, with powerful meaning. They form the mantra:

"Regularly eat a Variety of Whole foods."

This basic idea is used to capture how our evolutionary ancestors ate and what nutritional science has proven to be sound. I would not have needed to write this book if the Three Wisdoms were still part of our everyday vocabulary and understanding. The purpose of this book is to flesh out these concepts and give them meaning and practicality in your life.

Chapter 15

Wisdom 1
Regularity - timing is (almost) everything

The first basic rule or Wisdom of nutrition is to eat meals and snacks Regularly throughout the day. Not exactly rocket-science, but a much ignored principle.

No, you can't get by with only one meal, even if it is an excellent one. Your body requires regular intake of fuel as well as building and repair

> *"How can I eat so well and look so awful?"*

materials. Your body does not have a "coast" setting. If you wait too long to eat, you will slow down and, eventually, stop.

We all need balanced, healthy, nutrient-rich meals several times a day. I've counseled many patients who were trying to get by on one real meal a day. The usual scenario is that they have a reasonably good dinner every night, but skip breakfast and have a high-calorie, nutrient-poor lunch. This kind of eating pattern does not work for more than a few years before its weaknesses begin to reveal themselves.

Karen ate perfectly, but felt terrible

"How can I eat so well and look so awful?" Karen wanted so badly to feel and look better that she counted every calorie and every gram of carbohydrate, protein and fat. She'd started this one year before seeing me, after years of steadily gaining weight.

"I go to the gym five days a week. I work out hard for an hour to an hour and a half, without fail. How much more can I exercise?"

She was then 52 years old, thirty pounds over-weight and very frustrated. "Do I have to exercise seven days a week? I eat exactly the right amount of food. I never cheat. My husband thinks I'm a lunatic."

Every patient that sees me fills out a detailed food recall questionnaire on how much of various foods they eat every day. I've set it up so that I can quickly scan for problems such as too little protein, excess sweets, not enough vegetables, and other major nutritional factors. When I looked at Karen's, it appeared that she was doing what she said. Her protein, carbs and fat were in balance. She was taking in what seemed like the right amount of protein. However, the second part of the questionnaire revealed a glaring weakness.

"Karen," I said, "you do seem to be taking in a healthy balance of nutrients and not too much food. That's excellent. Now look at the second part of the questionnaire. You're not eating breakfast, only nibbling at lunch, then eating a large dinner. What this means is that you're starving yourself all day, when you need the energy, then eating this very healthy, but large, dinner right before you go to bed."

"I like to eat a normal meal when I'm with my husband," she replied.

"That's a great idea, but you won't have to worry so much about your total calories if you distributed them throughout the day."

I then went on to share with her a lot of the information you're about to read.

History and nutrition research show that people (and lab animals) do better with regular feedings. Regularity reduces weight gain (despite common weight-loss strategies) and improves overall health.

This does not necessarily mean a lot of food - only regular food. It might mean three meals per day. It might mean six nutritious snacks. Your biochemical individuality and activity level will determine the size and frequency.

Before the clock: Hunter-gatherer eating habits

Early food selection, when humans were developing the bodies and brains that would see them through to modern times, was from hunting and gathering. During this period of tens of thousands of years 99.9 percent of human genetic material was linked up and set in motion.

The food we were hunting and gathering was important for our development and survival. It was partially the reason our species survived while others died out. An integral part of that early diet was that people had few

"The pre-historic record clearly supports the principle of eating regularly."

resources for food storage. They ate as they gathered. Berries, vegetables, fruits, nuts, seeds, roots and other foraged foods were consumed as the foragers moved about. A woman passing a tree would pop buds in her mouth. If a flower known to be edible was available, it was part of the stew. If an animal was killed, the tribe ate their fill on the spot. Later, drying, salting and other simple methods of preservation were developed.

What is clear is that our body chemistry developed during a time that food was eaten regularly, even constantly throughout the day. Even if the kill of a large animal provided a feast, our ancestors would have been hungry a few hours later. For one thing, since 40 percent of caloric intake is used to generate heat, early peoples with primitive dwellings and clothing would have required the regular intake of food just to keep themselves warm.

What Modern Experts Say

The one thing that almost all diet and nutrition books agree upon is the need for regular meals. They may disagree on whether there should be three or eight meals per day, but no credible source advocates skipping meals.

Studies conducted on people who have successfully lost weight and kept it off show that these people almost always eat three or more meals per day and especially breakfast.

It's interesting that the one strategy for losing weight that no real nutrition expert advocates - skipping meals - is the one most commonly employed by the individual trying to lose pounds. It always backfires. Skipping meals is a desperate method that many people try, but it is rarely successful for losing weight over time.

Key Concept

Your body doesn't like to starve

As obvious as this is, it's ignored by most people and by thousands of weight-loss programs.

You do better with regular food intake. Sure, your body can deal with missing meals. It has created elaborate biochemical tricks, including slowing down your metabolism – the rate at which calories are burned - to preserve precious calories. If you only had 100 gallons of fuel to heat your house for the winter, you'd be cautious about how high you turned up the thermostat. Your body adopts this same strategy to lowered food intake by lowering your rate of metabolism (how many calories you burn).

The problem is, when you later increase your calorie intake your body doesn't always respond by increasing metabolism. The result of increased calories plus low metabolism is increased weight gain. Invariably, skipping meals leads to gaining weight. This is known as yoyo dieting – losing 10 pounds, then gaining 15. These dieters often end up much heavier than they would have been if they had never dieted.

The most successful weight-loss diets prescribe the regular intake of high quality foods. This keeps the metabolism revved up so that fat can be burned.

How many meals?

How many meals should you eat? The answer has to do with your unique biochemical individuality - a fancy way of saying that everyone is different.

It's an interesting statement about the power of genes to know that even though you and your neighbor have virtually the same genetic makeup, she may need to only eat three times per day while you need to eat six.

Finding your chow time

For my healthy patients, those who already feel good, I suggest they eat three healthy (although not large) meals per day and two snacks. This schedule mimics that of the hunter-gather and still fits into most people's work days with lunch and "coffee" breaks.

After a few weeks of the three-meal, two-snack schedule most people will know whether it's working for them. The best way to know is to take stock of how you're feeling when it's time for your next feeding. (I like the term "feeding" because it helps break people of the belief that meals are large and snacks consist of junk food. "Feedings" calls up the image of a baby who can eat whenever it desires.)

The time to eat is when you feel hungry, but not famished. If you wait too long, your blood sugar will drop, and your brain –the most sugar-sensitive organ – will not function well; your thoughts will become cloudy and your mood will suffer. Low blood sugar can result in irritability, anxiety, headache, sweaty palms, general weakness and craving for stimulants or sweets.

If sometime during the day you're excessively hungry or have low blood sugar symptoms, then something isn't right. There was probably a problem with your last feeding. It was either not a balanced meal or too much time had passed since you last ate.

Most people can go three hours without eating and not have a mental or physical melt-down. However, those with low blood sugar or diabetes may need to eat more often. On the other hand, it's not uncommon to find someone who does just fine on three meals daily without any ill effects or cravings. Again, you will know your feeding schedule is working for you if you feel good and don't find yourself frequently rummaging in the cookie jar. Or like Karen, you may find that excess weight is another indication that your feeding schedule is off.

Example of meal timing

There is no hard and fast rule on the "best" time to eat. The majority of people who work a typical 9 to 5 job will probably do well with a schedule similar to this:

- Somewhere between 7am & 8am: Breakfast.
- 10am: Light snack.
- 12noon: Lunch.
- Between 3pm & 4pm: Light snack.
- 6pm - 7pm: Dinner

Exact times, of course, will have to fit around work, sleep, exercise and errands. The time is not as important as how you feel.

If you've been eating at erratic times, try switching to

regular feeding times for a month and see if you don't feel better and your weight starts to drop.

In addition to blood sugar regulation, regular meal times also help set your daily circadian rhythm – your internal clock. Many people find they sleep better at night when their meals are regular.

By the way, Regular meals will not cause a dramatic weight loss. Look for a two to three pound per week loss. These low numbers can be frustrating if you're very overweight, but the loss will be steady until you reach equilibrium. If you're underweight, Regular meals will help you gain.

> *"Body fat percentage is found in research studies to be the most important indicator of health. A high percentage of fat increases your chances of cancer, stroke, heart disease and early death."*

Body fat percentage is found in research studies to be the most important indicator of health. A high percentage of fat increases your chances of cancer, stroke, heart disease and early death. Surprisingly, most doctors check cholesterol, yet few measure this far more important number – fat percentage. Healthy ranges for fat vary by age and sex. Your fat can be determined by fat calipers (which requires an experienced operator), a water emersion tank (an expensive test), or one of the newer home scales. Tanita® makes several scales for measuring weight, fat percentage and even water. (www.tanita.com)

Another excellent marker of health is your waist to hip ratio. Simply measure your waist at your belly button and your hips at their widest, and then divide the two. The ideal ratio for women is 0.8 and for men is below 0.95. This simple, low-cost measurement is an excellent predictor of risk for diabetes, heart disease and even early death.

Waist to Hip Ratio Chart		
Male	**Female**	**Health Risk Based on WHR**
0.95 or below	0.80 or below	Low Risk
0.96 to 1.0	0.81 to 0.85	Moderate Risk
1.0+	0.85+	High Risk

During weight loss, many people will find that first their percentage of fat will decline and then their total weight.

Modifying meal timing for blood sugar problems

Hypoglycemia

Low blood sugar, or hypoglycemia, is a common condition. It simply means that blood sugar levels have dropped too low to properly nourish the body and particularly the brain. Sugar is the major fuel for cells. Hypoglycemia most often results from a person consuming high amounts of refined carbohydrates and sugar. I know it seems like eating sugar would be the solution to low blood sugar, but the opposite is true. Your body works best on a steady, Regular intake of complex carbohydrates, protein and fat. Sugar is not a natural food for the body and disrupts measured energy release. (See Chapter 32.)

I find that my hypoglycemic patients need to be on a shorter leash – that is they need to eat more often than others. They do much better if they eat every one to three hours regardless of how they're feeling. Because when their blood sugar does drop, they quickly feel bad.

If they eat often, they can head off the low blood sugar symptoms and not find themselves in a situation where they have to rely on the kindness of our society to provide them with nutrition. If you're prepared to fortify yourself with a high-quality snack every hour or two, you're less likely to rely on junk food.

Sally: A Hypoglycemic Example

Let me illustrate hypoglycemia with a typical scenario. Sally was having increasing difficulty getting through her workday. "I work in a store where I have to know what four other people are doing and be nice to customers." Over the previous year she began having problems in the afternoon. She could hardly keep awake. "I find myself in the stock room looking for a place to hide and take a nap."

Her solution had been to drink a large cola with lunch followed by an after-lunch cup of coffee. This helped some, but around two o'clock she had to have another cola or coffee and something with chocolate from the snack bar. This kept her awake, but she was unable to focus on her work. Keeping track of inventory became difficult. "My computer screen sometimes looks like macramé." (Patients are so wonderfully descriptive!). But, worst of all, she found herself snapping at her customers. And, just to make matters worse, she had gained 12 pounds over the last year.

What is interesting to me was that she had let this go on for months without doing anything about it. She only went to see her MD after she'd had two episodes of irregular, rapid heart beats because that really scared her.

Her MD's solution was to prescribe a drug, Propranolol, which slowed her heart rate. Neither of them probed too deeply into why her heart was speeding up in the afternoon or, for that matter, what the side-effects might be of slowing down her heart. As it turns out, it wasn't good. Since starting the drug she felt light-headed often as well as lethargic and "spaced out" even more than before she started the prescription.

At a friend's suggestion, she reluctantly came to see me. After listening to her story, I asked about the rest of her diet, besides the cola, coffee and chocolate.

Breakfast: She didn't usually eat breakfast because she was "... too rushed in the morning to even think about eating."

Morning Break: "Coffee to get me in gear." Sometimes she ate a bagel or fruit.

Lunch: Lunches were eaten at one of a half-dozen restaurants she could rush to and back from in thirty minutes. Sandwiches, chicken teriyaki or pizza were her mainstays, since they could be ordered and eaten quickly.

Afternoon Break: I've already described the disaster of coffee, cola and chocolate.

Dinner: Too often she was too tired to cook, so she usually brought take-out home to her family. If she did cook, she often prepared pasta, chicken and a salad. Dinner was the most likely meal of the day to be balanced.

My diagnosis, one I've made hundreds of times, was afternoon hypoglycemia. She had all the classic symptoms - fatigue, irritability, craving caffeine and sugar, and sweaty palms.

The rapid heart rate was caused by a combination of excessive caffeine and her body's release of adrenal hormones. When a person's blood sugar drops, the brain, being the most sugar-dependant organ, knows about it pronto. The brain responds to hypoglycemia by sending crisis signals to the adrenal glands. Adrenal hormones will raise blood sugar, but will also cause nervousness, sweaty palms and an increased heart rate.

Her problem was not a deficiency of Propranolol to artificially slow her heart (and, incidentally, it also increases requirements for certain B vitamins) but a problem of irregular meals and insufficient nutrients. Her daily intake of protein may or may not have been adequate, but it was definitely not divided evenly throughout the day. She was also eating too much sugar and starch.

Sally's Blood Sugar Prescription

My advice to Sally was for her to start eating three balanced meals and four balanced snacks every day. I also prescribed vitamins and minerals that would help her to control her blood sugar.

A week later she reported to me that she was already feeling better, but that she was still craving sweets and caffeine in the afternoon. I had not told her to eliminate caffeine, only to start the process of cutting back. I knew that as her energy improved, she would no longer have the craving.

Because she continued to have afternoon symptoms, we modified her program to have her eat every two hours. As I explained to her, "It doesn't have to be much, but it does have to contain protein and fat as well as complex carbohydrates." I also added, "You will feel progressively better over the next six to twelve months. In the meantime, I suggest you eat every two hours for at least three months. After that, you can try eating every three hours. If you feel alright, continue eating every three hours for six months, then check back with me."

A Life-saving Concept:
CARRY EMERGENCY FOODS WITH YOU AT ALL TIMES

Nuts, seeds, cheese, hard-boiled eggs, protein bars or shakes are all foods that travel well. Do not leave yourself at the mercy of vending machines, take-out counters, deli foods or convenience stores. They often do not carry the quality food you need.

After nine to twelve months of Regularly eating every 1 to 3 hours, you will have recovered enough that you will not need to be so strict about your eating schedule. Until then, you will feel better and recover faster if you follow this program.

Of course we also spoke at length about what foods were best for her to eat and those to avoid as described in Chapter 17, Wholeness.

Sally, like most of my patients, was rewarded many times over for her efforts. In addition to feeling better at work and not getting fired for her attitude, she lost weight and had more energy in the evening. That energy transferred into more quality time spent with her family.

Diabetes

Diabetics tend to have high blood sugar and trouble regulating their insulin. The same prescription that is good for hypoglycemics – regular small feedings through the day – is also good for diabetics.

It has been discovered that the worst thing for diabetics is to have spikes in their blood sugar. These spikes set off a cascade of events that predispose them to heart disease, stroke, blindness and poor wound healing.

Both Type 1 and Type 2 diabetics gain better control over their blood sugar if they avoid irregular large meals. For more on hypoglycemia and diabetes, see Chapter 32.

Is breakfast necessary?

This has to be one of the most-asked questions by people trying to change their diet.

The simple answer is "Yes".

Besides being the advice of millions of moms, there is a plethora of scientific research to support the benefits of breakfast.

What better time to "break your fast" than in the morning when you're preparing to be alert and active? Eating breakfast makes both common sense and biochemical sense.

In one interesting study, two groups were fed the exact same diet and number of calories. The difference was that one group ate most of their food in the early part of the day and the other group ate the bulk of their food in the later part of the day. The early eaters lost weight. The late eaters gained weight. This is not surprising when you consider that it's in the daytime that you need your calories and not in the evening when you should be resting, not digesting.

Numerous studies have shown that eating breakfast helps patients gain muscle and lose fat. This is what made the difference for Karen. She was able to lose weight and feel better by cutting down on her dinner portion and increasing her nutrients and calories at breakfast and lunch. This simple change in timing increased her energy and reduced her weight, although her total number of calories actually went up!

Ken: "But doctor…"

Ken, a middle-aged Microsoft manager who consulted with me about his newly-diagnosed diabetes, asked me a common question. "I've been skipping breakfast for years, why should I change now?"

Like most patients who ask me this question, Ken was no longer functioning at the high level that he was use to. In fact, he was worried that he might lose his job.

I responded, "Your eating habits worked when you were young and had more reserves. Now your ability to regulate glucose is not working as well as it once did. In my experience, your condition will get worse unless you do something about it. Right now your glucose is only modestly high, but it will continue to go up if you don't make some simple changes now."

Yes, I have patients who skip breakfast and eat poorly through the day and still feel fine. They're usually under 30 years old and it is sometimes difficult to convince them that what they're doing will have long-term consequences. I can only tell them my experience, share with them how their distant ancestors ate, and what the research shows: you're better off eating Regular meals, including breakfast.

I have on rare occasions met someone who is over fifty, in excellent condition, and doesn't eat breakfast. Viva la difference and isn't biochemical individuality amazing? However, this is extremely rare. In my experience, the ones who claim this (almost exclusively men) are in denial about how they really feel. Sure, you can cover up a lot of bad feelings with a caffeinated soda or strong cup of coffee, but not forever.

Ken responded well to eating regular meals. He'd been worried about his job because his employer was making cutbacks and he'd been performing poorly due to swings in his blood sugar. Within days he regained his energy and clarity of thought and was not part of the next round of layoffs.

Not hungry at meal time?

If you find yourself not feeling hungry at snack or meal time, the answer is not to skip that feeding. Again, by looking to the last feeding, you will probably discover the answer. Usually the problem is that the last meal or snack was too large. Remember, the plan is to eat regular **small** meals and snacks.

If not being hungry is a persistent problem for you, consult a naturopathic physician to find out if you have an underlying health issue. Hormonal, digestive and other problems can interfere with a person's appetite or make them feel full when they haven't been eating.

It's a common mistake to wait until you're feeling

hungry before looking for food. Healthy people may be able to get away with it, but those with blood sugar problems should not do this. They need to eat at regular intervals.

Can't stomach breakfast?

Occasionally I have patients who complain that they can't eat breakfast because they feel queasy or nauseated in the morning.

It is abnormal to not feel hungry after an overnight fast of eight to twelve hours. While your stomach may be telling you not to eat, the cells of your brain, liver, kidneys, and rest of your body are in need of nutrients. The belly is saying no while the cells are saying "Feed me!"

One common reason for this problem is eating late the night before. Protein and fat-rich foods are the worst offenders. The remedy for late-night hunger is to eat better earlier in the day. As you shift to eating healthier meals and snacks throughout the day, you will find yourself less hungry in the late evening. Once you break yourself of late-night eating, you'll feel better, and hungrier, the next morning. Cutting out late-night snacks is also an excellent way to lose weight.

Many of my patients find that a breakfast protein shake sits well in their tummy.

If changing your eating pattern doesn't help your morning appetite, consult a naturopathic physician.

Regularity summary

Regularity is a word that represents the concept of eating regularly through the day. It is a critical part of the three-legged nutritional stool on which good health sits. Just like Karen, you could be eating a good diet of just the right calories, but if you're not spreading those calories throughout the day and especially at breakfast, then your health and weight will likely suffer.

Most people do best with three meals and two snacks per day. The exact times will vary, depending on your schedule and metabolism.

Diabetic and hypoglycemic patients may need to eat more often – for instance three or four light snacks instead of two. Meal timing is probably the most important thing most people with blood sugar problems – high or low - can do for themselves.

Your feedings should not be large unless you are performing heavy manual labor or extreme exercise. This is especially true of dinner. A big dinner and a big easy chair are big reasons for big people.

Skipping meals will not help you lose weight but, in fact, will do quite the opposite.

Make Regularity a part of your eating life and watch how your health improves.

Chapter 16

Wisdom 2

Variety - It is the spice of life

Variety refers to eating a wide assortment of foods. It is a Wisdom because it is supported by the historic record and by modern science. Unfortunately, it is not a Regular part of most people's eating habits.

As a test, ask yourself which carbohydrates you've eaten this week. Many people could name only one, usually wheat. But what about corn, potatoes, yams, millet, barley, lentils, and squash? These are all mostly carbohydrates as are most fruits and vegetables. If you named a number of them, then you're already incorporating Variety in your diet.

> "Eating a Variety of different foods is a simple concept, but it's difficult for many of us to implement. We tend to get into the habit of eating the same foods day after day."

Although we have a huge variety of fruits, vegetables, grains and other starches available in our supermarkets, most of us tend to stay with familiar foods.

The same thing happens with proteins. Some people limit themselves to beef and cheese. But turkey, lamb, fish, nuts, yogurt, quinoa, eggs and beans all contain significant amounts of protein.

It's not just the fast-food people who lack variety. I've had vegetarian patients who rely on soy as their only protein source.

Because our supermarkets import foods from around the world, we have more choices, but too many of us eat the same thing day after day all year around. Few people take advantage of the wide variety of foods that are available to them.

The Paleolithic Grocery Store

It is estimated that ancient hunter-gatherers ate approximately 200 varieties of foods. Today the average is 20. You may know people who eat fewer. A fast-food addict will only be eating wheat (the bun), potatoes (French fries), beef (hamburger), processed cheese (cheeseburger), lettuce and tomatoes. What's that? Six foods? Even if you add a breakfast sandwich (eggs and more wheat), and the soy that's used as a filler in the beef, that's only eight foods. No wonder these people never feel satisfied.

The hunter-gatherer was in constant contact with a multitude of foods - and therefore nutrients. Some of the foods in their varied diet we no longer consider foods. Wild flowers are packed with nutrients that few of us have ever experienced. Chewing on flower buds was a source of micro-nutrients, flavonoids and oils which are often deficient in modern diets. For instance, quercetin, a flavonoid that is now being used successfully in capsule form to treat allergies, is found in high concentrations in organic vegetables and the bark of trees. Have you had your bark today?

Cooking and chewing on bones and tendons provided important nutrients for our ancestors' joints and connective tissues. Now some people substitute a capsule of chondroitin sulfate or gelatin for their arthritis.

The constellation of nutrients that was part of the hunter-gatherer's daily foraging experience is lost to us. Researchers believe, for instance, that we consume one tenth as much potassium as our ancient ancestors and ten times more sodium. This reversal of traditional potassium and sodium intake contributes to high blood pressure. And it is believed that most of us take in far fewer of the other minerals than our ancestors.

Unfortunately, to a large degree we don't even know all that we've lost. Thousands of species of animals and plants have become extinct. Some of the nutrients have been bred out of foods in order to make their taste more appealing or because qualities such as size, shape and bruise-resistance are more valued by the food industry.

It makes nutritional sense for you to add more Variety into your diet.

Variety big and small

Food can be broadly broken down into two categories: Macronutrients and Micronutrients

- **Macronutrients**: Macro means big and refers to proteins, carbohydrates and fats.

- **Micronutrients**: Micro means small and refers to vitamins, minerals, antioxidants and other microscopic food factors in the diet.

The Wisdom of Variety is applied to both macro- and micronutrients. The best meals and snacks incorporate proteins, carbohydrates, fats and a broad assortment of micronutrients.

Macronutrient Variety

When choosing something to eat, it's always helpful to ask

yourself, "What are the protein, carb and fat in this feeding?" This process takes microseconds of brain time, but may add years of longevity to your life.

Let's look at a few common examples:

> It's three o'clock in the afternoon and you know that if you don't have a healthy snack soon, you'll dip into the office M&M stash. Your choices are an apple and jar of almonds. Which do you choose? If you remember Variety, you'll go for both. The apple supplies mostly carbohydrates (like all fruits except avocados) and the almonds supply protein and fats (like most nuts and seeds). "But that's too much food" you protest. It may very well be more than you want to eat, so cut the apple in half or quarters and only have a handful of almonds. If you're following the first Wisdom, Regularity, you will never be in a situation where you feel compelled to eat a lot of food.

Next example:

> It's breakfast time and you love to blend up fruit smoothies. There's nothing wrong with that if you remember that fruit is mostly carbohydrate, so you need to add a protein and a fat to your blend. If you add a protein powder such as whey, soy or rice protein, that provides the protein, but you'll still need some fat. Flaxseeds or flaxseed oil, fish oil (the best brands have practically no fish flavor), coconut oil, or even a splash of olive oil will round off your shake.

I could go on with examples. The bottom line is that each time you eat, take a couple of seconds to assess your options of macronutrient variety: protein, starch and fat.

Micronutrient Variety

The greatest abundance of micronutrients comes from fruits, berries and vegetables. Variety comes from eating many different kinds of foods.

Advertisers will tout the latest miracle antioxidant fruit (usually imported at great expense from a tropical climate) but the best way to insure you're taking in the most powerful anti-cancer and anti-aging micronutrients is to eat a variety of different foods.

An easy way to add micro variety is to add color. The color of a fruit or vegetable reflects the kinds of micronutrients contained in that plant. Look for reds, yellows, blues, oranges and even different shades of green.

Lack of variety – modern consequences

Does it really matter that we no longer eat several different varieties of grains and potatoes, dozens of different vegetables or a microscopic amount of an obscure plant alkaloid found in cedar buds? There is scientific evidence that limiting our food choices with mono-eating may be causing a number of health problems.

Variety increases nutrients

No single food has all the nutrients you need. By increasing the variety in your diet, you increase the likelihood of ingesting the greatest number of nutrients.

Variety increases your complement of carbs, protein, and fat. A balance of the three helps regulate blood sugar and hormone levels.

Each food has its strengths. For instance, wheat has more protein than potatoes. But potatoes have more vitamin

C. Quinoa and millet have almost twice as much protein as wheat, yet are often overlooked by those who lack variety.

Proteins are made of chains of amino acids. Twenty amino acids combine to build all of the proteins in your body. Foods vary in the amount and types of amino acids they contain. As a rule, animal proteins have more amino acids than plant proteins. Combining two different foods, like beans and grains, increases the number of amino acids available to you.

Vitamin and mineral levels also vary among foods. Potatoes have more vitamin C than wheat. Nuts have more zinc than grains. In addition, some varieties of potatoes are higher in vitamin C while others are higher in potassium. Salmon species vary greatly in the relative amounts of protein and fat and have far more fat – the good kind - than white fish.

Micronutrients such as flavonoids, many of which have only been discovered in the last 40 years, vary greatly between plants and even in the same plant at different times of the year. The orange vegetable has different flavonoids than the yellow and red fruits.

I could go on. The point is, by eating a Variety of foods you increase the likelihood that you're taking in all of the nutrients you body grew up with, evolutionarily speaking. What your ancestors consumed is likely to contribute to your health.

Variety reduces food sensitivities

Another reason to eat more variety besides nutrient content is to avoid food sensitivities. Eating the same food excessively is associated with developing allergies or food intolerances.

A full discussion of food sensitivities is beyond the scope of this book. But, simply stated, people tend to develop sensitivities to foods that they ingest on a regular basis. That is why the most commonly eaten foods including dairy, wheat, corn, and soy, are the most common allergens.

You may wonder why soy allergy would be so common since most Americans do not choose to eat soybeans, tofu, miso and other soy products on a regular basis. Soy, however, is a common additive in processed foods, baby food, and is used to "stretch" ground hamburger meat. Likewise, corn derivatives are common in processed foods.

A food allergy or sensitivity happens after a person is exposed to a food. Their immune system mistakes the food for a harmful substance and manufactures antibodies against it. It's similar to the process by which we develop immunity to a particular flu virus. Once exposed, the immune system makes antibodies which kill off that same virus if it comes around again.

With food, once the antibodies are in your system, they will react every time you eat that food. This could be sneezing, a runny nose, itchy skin, digestive distress or even mental confusion. If however, you don't eat that food for a while, the antibody production will diminish or cease all together. You may then be able to eat that food again occasionally without having a reaction.

Other food reactions can be triggered by things other than antibodies. Although not well researched, some people have non-antibody food reactions. The process is not completely understood but what research does exist relates these reactions to changes in digestion.

> By simply rotating your intake of all foods, you reduce exposure, antibody production and reactive symptoms. In order to rotate your intake of foods you must introduce the second Wisdom - Variety.

Symptoms of food sensitivity

Reactions to foods can include a wide variety of symptoms: rashes, runny nose, itchy eyes, indigestion, gas, bloating, asthma, joint pain, headache, fatigue, gallstones, dyslexia, attention deficit hyperactive disorder, and more. (See Chapter 36 for more information on food sensitivities.)

Variety increases your sensual pleasure

I encourage my patients to eat a variety of foods because this exposes them to a greater number of smells and tastes. A varied diet is a treat for your senses and a party of sensory delights.

Paleolithic people must have been bombarded with a cornucopia of tastes and smells that they learned to distinguish from one another. The pleasure of smelling and tasting foods is part of the process of eating. Body chemicals such as enzymes and hormones are released in response to these stimuli.

One of the consequences of eating a limited diet is that our children are denied the opportunity of developing their sense of smell and taste.

I believe that part of the reason so many people overeat is because on some subliminal level their body desires more tastes and smells than they are exposing themselves to.

The food industry smothers us in salt and sugar, salt and sugar, salt and sugar. They know through extensive research (if only they put as much energy into increasing the nutrient value!) that our tongues are acutely sensitive to these two tastes. Our ancestors' survival depended on being able to distinguish tastes, especially sugar and salt. Now we're being kept taste-prisoners of these two and denied the pleasure of other tastes.

This lack of variety of tastes and smells is, in my opinion, part of the reason so many people eat as if they're starving. The standard American diet lacks the array of subtle stimuli that trigger satisfaction in our appetite centers. When a meal is rich in flavor, it's enjoyed more. A flavorful meal is generally eaten slower and provides a truly satisfying culinary experience.

Variety is good for the environment

Not only does variety help us individually, but it helps the environment. The farming industry has reduced the number and the varieties of foods it produces. For instance, there used to be dozens of types of wheat and corn available. Since the 1940's there are 80 to 90 percent fewer varieties being grown.

Agribusiness and the practice of planting single varieties of a crop (mono-culturing) have dramatically reduced our choices. It is easier and cheaper to plant millions of acres of a single type of potato. The most popular potato currently being grown is the one that lends itself to slicing and deep-fat frying in fast-food outlets. (Can they really be called restaurants?) Because of potato mono-culturing, there is currently a blight attacking millions of acres of potatoes around the world.

No, this book wasn't written a hundred years ago in Ireland. This is occurring today in the U.S. Huge fields of potatoes are being ploughed under because the blight has made them unfit for consumption. This is analogous to the Irish potato famine in which blight caught hold of the single variety of potato being grown at the time. Nature is naturally diversified. When you harvest only one variety of a plant, various pests have an easier time mounting an attack.

Today, millions of dollars are being spent in combating the current explosion of blight. Chemical poisons are being mixed and applied as you read this. Potatoes that are blight-resistant are being bio-engineered. The newest technologies in gene-splicing and cloning are drafted into the fight against blight. Unfortunately, little attention is being paid to the nutrient value of the single type of potato.

The truth is that all of this money, time and technological effort are unnecessary. The remedy for blight is already known. The problem is that agribusiness won't accept the known cure for blight. The solution is to stop mono-culturing and to grow more varieties on smaller parcels of land. By adding variety to the field, the blight can no longer take over and destroy all the potatoes. Blight grows stronger when there is only one variety of potatoes and is weaker when there are many. Without variety, plant diseases are better able to succeed in spreading.

Some varieties of plants - potatoes in this example - are more resistant to certain infections. By planting a wide variety of a plant, as is done in organic gardening, the farmer decreases the possibility of total crop destruction.

The same strategy applies to wheat and other grains. There used to be hundreds of varieties, and now only a few are commonly grown.

Anti-Terrorist Farming

Mono-culturing also makes our farm crops more vulnerable to biological terrorism. The Soviet Union, during the Cold War, experimented with a strain of fungus that was lethal to wheat. Iraq is believed to have also experimented with food terrorism.

If a strain of wheat-killing fungus were released into the mid-western United States today, millions of acres would be devastated. Our crops are vulnerable because of mono-cropping. When only one variety of wheat is grown, a terrorist agent can spread and destroy easily.

If, on the other hand, there are many different types of wheat being grown or, better yet, many different crops are companion-planted, the destructive element will more likely be confined to a smaller area. Organic farmers plant in this manner.

Adding variety to your life

In order to add variety to your diet, it is necessary to reduce repetitive eating. Repetitive eating means eating the same food day after day.

Reducing repetitive eating begins with taking inventory of your diet. Wheat and dairy are common examples of foods people eat every day, often several times a day. Other common repetitive foods are corn, beef and chicken. Vegetarians tend to eat a lot of soy and brown rice. Oranges are the most commonly eaten fruit and tomatoes are the most common vegetable.

Some of my patients, when first learning how to add variety to their diet, write out their foods on a calendar. This way they can see plainly which foods they are eating and if they have fallen into repetitively eating the same food.

Once you have a clear idea of what you're eating now, there are three methods for adding variety.

Eating with the seasons

The seasons of the year help you achieve variety. Shop for what's grown locally and in season. Your genetic ancestors, the hunter-gatherers, would not have eaten out of season foods. In-season foods are at their nutritional peak and are less expensive.

Of course this is not possible if you live in a severe northern climate. You don't have a choice but to eat foods grown in other places. The one choice you do have is sprouts (see Chapter 46). Sprouts are grown indoors with just seeds and water. Organic seeds are available for sprouting.

Less severe northern climates like Washington and Oregon are able to grow vegetables all year around. No matter where you live, seek out ways to avoid aviation foods – those flown in from thousands of miles away. If you can't completely eliminate imported foods, at least strive for variety. Even foods imported from warmer climates will change with the seasons. Generally speaking, whatever is in abundance or on sale is what is in season.

Many of my patients find that joining a Community Supported Agriculture (CSA) program is an excellent way to encourage variety. They pay a monthly price to have a local farmer, usually organic, deliver fresh vegetables. Each week a bag appears on their porch, or at a convenient drop location, overflowing with seasonal fresh fruits and vegetables. You don't only get produce you are familiar with, but the adventure and health benefits of figuring out what to do with an exotic new vegetable are worth their weight in health. CSAs are also good for the farmer because they encourage more organic farming! To find a CSA program in your area, visit www.localharvest.org/csa.

Avoidance method

You can also add variety to your meals by simply identifying a food, or several foods, that you eat every day, and avoiding them for a while. "Avoidance" in this case really means reducing your consumption to two or three times per week.

Once you've reduced your consumption of a food you'll want to come up with a substitute. Look for a food in the same category – carbohydrate, protein, or fat.

For instance, if you've been eating wheat 2 to 3 times a day, you'll want to find another carbohydrate such as rice, beans, potatoes, yams, millet, broccoli, rutabagas, etc. Fruit, at certain meals or snacks, can become a substitute for wheat crackers, bread, croissants, muffins, and the like. If it's a protein, such as cheese, that you're eating too often, then look for ways of substituting fish, tofu, turkey, eggs, nuts, and other protein-rich foods.

Some people eat the same vegetables day after day. Ask the produce person at your market which vegetables are grown locally. Again, whatever is in season will tend to be less expensive and even on sale.

Avoidance can be particularly difficult with dairy and wheat as they are so ubiquitous in our culture. Fortunately, in the case of wheat, non-wheat cereals, noodles, crackers and even breads are available. If you're a sandwich eater, think of creative ways to make sandwiches using corn tortilla wraps or, my favorite, the potato sandwich. Slice open a baked potato or yam, hot or cold, and add your favorite sandwich ingredients - being careful to avoid repetition, of course.

Category method

Okay, you're hungry. A healthy way to go about satisfying your hunger is to first think about the major food groups – carbs, protein and fats. Each meal or snack should have something from all three groups. This blend helps stabilize blood sugar, neurotransmitters and hormones.

Now think about adding Variety to the major food groups. An excellent method of adding variety to your diet is by categorizing the foods you consume by food group. Dividing foods into carbohydrates, proteins and fats helps you evaluate what you're eating repetitively and enables you to substitute a new food.

Carbohydrates

Carbohydrates, or starches, are the most abundant foods we eat. A common problem in the U.S. is that many people eat only one food from this category - wheat.

You may be eating wheat every day and often several times a day in the form of bread, cereal, muffins, pasta and baked goods. This is a concern because you are denying yourself the health-giving nutrition of other carbohydrates. Also, wheat is one of the most common allergenic foods. And remember that processed foods are a common place for wheat to hide.

The remedy is to introduce other foods in this

category such as potatoes, rice, millet, barley, quinoa, corn, sweet potatoes and oats, to name a few.

It is important to remember that vegetables and fruit are, for the most part, also carbohydrates. You don't need to have grain-based starches in your diet at all. Before about 9000 years ago - a relatively short time in human evolution - grains were not a major part of the diet.

I recommend that my patients try, as much as possible, to substitute vegetables and fruits for grains. This can help sedentary people cut calories. Those of you who need the extra calories may need some form of grain, but it need not be wheat.

Hunter-gathers ate wild vegetables, roots and fruits as their major carbohydrate source. Later, with the development of agriculture (and animal domestication) grains became a staple part of the diet. Some researchers believe that the grain-based diet was the start of many human illnesses. For instance, arthritis has become more common since the introduction of grains. Anthropologists have also shown that human height diminished after the introduction of grains. The skeletons of many of our ancient ancestors are comparable in size to modern humans. Height diminished after the introduction of large-scale agriculture. Humans did not begin returning to their former stature until the introduction of iron tools and other improvements in agriculture increased calorie consumption.

Some researchers point to the addictive nature of grains, especially wheat. Wheat stimulates the release of endorphins which are mood enhancing. This can be dangerous for those who tend to be depressed or fatigued. The temporary surge of feeling good can lead to addictive behavior with ups and downs in mood and energy. Better to find the cause of the underlying problem and fix it rather than relying on wheat as a drug.

With my patients I emphasize vegetables and fruit over grains as sources of carbohydrates. This is especially true of low-energy expenditure office workers. They generally do not need the extra calories of grains.

To add variety to your fruits and vegetables, think color. White fruits like apples and bananas are good, but don't forget your blue, red, and yellow fruits. The same is true for vegetables: green is fantastic, but you'll find a rainbow of colors available when you start looking.

Protein

Protein is another category of food that can be subdivided. Dairy is a commonly overeaten protein food. It is also, statistically speaking, the most allergic food.

To add variety to your proteins, substitute other protein foods such as black, red, or white beans or one of the many kinds of other beans. Nuts of all kinds contain healthy proteins. Various fish species – not just tuna, tuna, tuna – add spice to meals. Other great protein choices are organically-raised eggs, chicken and other meats.

I like the style of cooking found in Southeast Asia, France and Mediterranean countries I've visited where they often use protein as a garnish, such as long beans with a hint of shrimp or other seafood.

Fats

While your typical grocery shelf is over-stocked with several brands of low-quality soy, corn and vegetable oils, there are many other quality oils to choose from. You may have to seek out a specialty market or health-food store to find other tasty selections.

Nuts provide an excellent array of good-quality oils. Sesame oil can be found in Asian markets. Extra-virgin olive oil is available in many better-quality supermarkets. Flax seed oil, borage oil and avocados are also excellent sources of good-quality oil.

The oils I recommend are more difficult to find, but you only need to buy them once a month or less. They should be kept under refrigeration to retard rancidity, a common problem with oils. Adding the contents of a natural vitamin E capsule to the bottle of oil is an excellent extra defense against rancidity.

Limit vegetable oils such as corn, canola and soybean. Absolutely avoid trans-fatty acids and hydrogenated oils. (See Chapters 9 and 10 for more on fats.)

Summary of Variety

Your ancestors evolved on a Variety of foods. They were not one-stop shoppers or supporters of monotonous rows of the same crop. They dug, plucked, picked and chewed hundreds of different varieties of plants and animals. Modern people who eat more Variety tend to be healthier.

Variety decreases the possibility of turning food into your enemy in the form of an allergy or sensitivity. When you select a Variety of foods, you support greater plant diversity and healthy farming practices, as well as contributing to your own good health.

Expose yourself to a greater variety of vitamins, minerals, proteins, fats and other nutrients by being more adventurous in your eating.

When shopping and eating, pause to think about Macro and Micro Variety: Protein, carbohydrates, fats and micronutrients. The more color in your diet, the better.

Variety is more than the spice of life; it is a fundamental requirement for healthy eating.

Chapter 17

Wisdom 3

Wholeness – from whole to wholesome

Wholeness is another principal concept of a healthy eating program. Whole is what your food should be. Regularity and Variety, the other core concepts of this program, are what you do with Whole foods. Simply stated, nutrition in a nutshell is eating Whole foods, Regularly and in great Variety. If you can remember "Regularly eat a Variety of Whole foods," you are well on your way to cutting through the media confusion, avoiding diet fads and knowing what to shop for.

What is a whole food?

The dictionary definitions of "Whole" are helpful and illuminating: "Comprising the full quantity or amount; Complete; Undivided; Not fractional; Not broken, damaged, or impaired; Pertaining to all aspects of human nature (e.g. "Education for the whole person"); A thing complete in itself or comprising all its parts or elements; A unitary system; Uninjured or unharmed."

Healthy nutrition means applying the above definitions

to food. When you eat foods that are not broken, fractured, damaged or otherwise impaired, then you are eating foods that are complete with the full quantity of nutrients. These are known as whole foods.

Whole, wholistic and wholeness are words you need to keep in mind when thinking about meal planning, shopping, cooking and eating out. I prefer "wholistic" over "holistic" because I am not referring to "holes" in apples, but to "whole" apples.

Three Characteristics of Whole Foods

The definition of "Whole" describes exactly how food should be eaten. The best foods are complete; not broken, damaged or impaired. They contain the full quantity of their parts or elements. A healthy food is a food that is uninjured or unharmed.

I take the term literally and in its broadest interpretation. The healthiest meals, as I'll explain more in depth later in this section, are the ones that are as close as possible to what your hunter-gatherer ancestors ate. Wholeness can be summarized as food that is:

1. **Fresh**
2. **Organic**
3. **Un-processed**

Let's discuss each of these in detail starting with Fresh.

Wholeness Principle One: Freshness

Fresh-faced Foods: Why Freshness Counts

The term "Fresh off the vine," even in this age of agribusiness and supermarkets, is still recognizable. While few of our foods today are truly fresh - unless you have a backyard garden - we still seem to know instinctively that the very best foods are fresh off a vine, a tree, a bush, an herb, or pulled from the earth. This is, of course, how our ancestors ate everything.

For a food to be truly whole, it must be fresh.

Before refrigeration, vacuum-packing, warehouses, trucks and even agriculture, food was eaten "Living fresh." It was plucked fresh from where it grew or - hold your stomach - sliced right from the animal and, without much ado, tossed into the mouth.

Freshness is part of Wholeness because a fresh food is more complete in vitamins, minerals and other nutrition factors.

While I'm not recommending ripping the pounding heart from inside a bison and passing it around at your next family meal, there are modern ways to insure you consume the powerful, health-building nutrients that are found in fresh live food.

If it Ain't Living, it's Rotting

If you think about it, you realize that as soon as any food is separated from its life-source, the earth, it begins to decay. Dead food rots. We can slow down that rotting process by refrigeration, freezing, drying, salting, canning or otherwise restricting heat, air, light and moisture, but these are merely delaying tactics. The food will eventually become compost.

The spoilage of food means a process by which vitamins, minerals and other food factors are lost. Fats go rancid. Proteins break down. Mold, bacteria, maggots, viruses and worms do what they've done for millions of years, compost food back into the earth. To borrow from Bob Dylan, food that isn't busy being born is busy dying.

What passes as fresh today

We've come a long way from our early ancestors and we've moved a long way from our food sources. You have no need to bother growing corn in your state when the world is so small it can be driven in from Kansas in a couple of days. Idaho potatoes are only a few interstates away from your grocery store. Tons of Guatemalan strawberries can be packed onto a cargo plane. Jet fuel provides us with Alaskan salmon.

Today, food in the U.S. travels an average of 1300 miles before it reaches a consumer. The Interstate Highway System and even your local airport are more a part of the food chain than the acreage around most cities. Those formerly rural lands have been turned into industrial parks and suburbs. Food growing is being pushed farther away from where people eat it.

The encroachment of housing developments has started a modern "range war." Instead of cattle ranchers against sheep herders, the battle is between the few

"Where I live in Seattle, much of the local farm land that is rich with millions of years of volcanic minerals has been covered over by technology companies and high-end housing. What little remaining farmland there is has been converted from growing food to growing grass which is rolled up and sold as instant lawn."

remaining farmers and the local soccer association that sees every open field as an athletic opportunity. Parents seem to value teaching their children sportsmanship over nutritional sense. They don't understand the health implications of their children eating oranges that were picked green in Florida weeks before being peeled. (They also don't know that the peel has been dyed orange.)

The ravages of time

The sooner you eat a food after it has been picked, the better. As a general rule, it's best not to eat green leafy vegetables that are over a few days old. You might find them filling, but they are not very nutritious.

We live on nutrients. The reason for eating well is to live well. If our food is not fresh, it is not well. It has been devalued. The reason for us to eat has wasted away.

Keeping it fresh

In this era of a supposedly shrinking world in which everyone and everything, including every sort of food, is just hours away, it can be frustratingly difficult to find fresh food. As the world has gotten "smaller" the distance between an ear of fresh sweet corn and your mouth has become greater.

There are strategies that can keep you in touch with fresh, nutrient-rich produce.

Grow your own

The ideal system for having fresh fruits and vegetables is to grow your own. Home growing on small plots of land and even in window sills can be very productive. It is estimated that 70 percent of the produce eaten in Hong Kong is grown in this fashion. Most United States cities have far more cultivatable land than population-dense Hong Kong.

A well-organized backyard garden can be used to grow enough fresh produce to supply an entire family with fresh vegetables from Spring until Fall. Many states have mild enough climates to grow a winter crop of luscious greens.

Once organized, a garden takes little time to maintain, gives family members a collective project, is a safe nature classroom for children, provides a space for meditation, and is a great excuse to exercise, especially stretching.

There are many excellent books on home gardening. It's important to find one that applies to your climate.

On a smaller scale, home sprouting can be a delicious way to cheaply supply one of the most vitamin-packed foods you can find. (See Chapter 46 on Sprouting.)

Farmers' Markets

Many cities are now supporting farmers markets where local small farmers can sell the fruits of their labors directly to the consumer. In Seattle, besides the bustling downtown Pike Street Market (said to be the oldest continuously operating farmers' market in the U.S.) there are several community markets that are open on different days of the week.

The United States is still way behind Europe, Asia, Mexico and, now that I think of it, most every other city, town and village in the world, but access to local farmer's markets is improving. It's always a happy, delicious and colorful experience to find the local market in Arel, France, Chaing Mai, Thailand or wherever I'm traveling.

Part of the problem for U.S. cities is that the sprawling suburbs have pushed the farmland to inconvenient distances. In Seattle, some farmers have to come in by ferry or drive across the Cascade Mountains. The produce is picked early on the morning of the market, stacked in trucks and driven for hours. These fruits and vegetables, while not right out of the garden, are still fresher than those available in most grocery chains.

Green Shopping

Another approach to finding fresh food is to become what I call a Green Shopper. This means buying your produce daily or at least several times per week. I'm reminded of the era when small "mom-and-pop" stores were conveniently located within walking distance in every neighborhood. Although on the decline, this system of Green Shopping still functions in most of the world. This is one of the reasons that most of the world is healthier than Americans.

Daily shopping is the best, but many people find this impossible. Even if you have the time, there is often too much traffic or not enough parking or no public transportation. However, you might be able to shop three days a week at farmer's markets or your local organic produce market. Find out which days local produce is delivered and make those your shopping days.

Shopping can be surprisingly quick if you're just picking up vegetables and fruit and not wading through long aisles of canned and packaged food. You also qualify for the express check-out. Green shopping can be done in as little as ten minutes.

Produce Delivery

Another option your community might have is a produce-subscription service, or CSA. (See also Chapter 16 on Variety.) You pay a monthly fee to have seasonal vegetables and fruits delivered to you by a local organic farmer each week. This is the produce equivalent of the old-time milkman.

You pay a little more, of course, for the convenience, but it's a great way of getting the freshest produce and decreasing the stress of shopping.

The major complaint about this system is that you don't always get what you want. When the growing season for peas is over, your supply is cut off. On the other hand, this can also be viewed as an advantage. You are forced into eating a Variety of foods you might otherwise not be drawn to. Suddenly you'll be standing in front of a stove with a hand full of rutabagas remembering that Variety is one of the Three Wisdoms.

Preserved Foods

Fresh is best. It gives you the highest quality nutrition. There are times, however, when fresh isn't available.

An obvious limitation on eating fresh foods is weather. The cold of Northern climates tends to freeze out winter gardens. Although many people do live in zones where vegetables will grow all year long, most people don't winter garden. It's a shame, but this is how things are now. In winter most people will rely on a higher percentage of preserved foods.

Preserved food is sometimes necessary. You should be aware that all preservation techniques reduce, to some degree, the quality of the food. It's important to select the foods that retain the most nutritional quality. Food has been preserved in various ways for thousands of years. Canning, drying, salting and freezing are common techniques for keeping foods for prolonged periods of time.

Fermentation and pickling are other ways of storing food. You may not think you eat fermented foods unless you realize that cheese, yogurt, kefir and buttermilk are fermented, as are sauerkraut, pickles, and Korean kimchee.

Recent anthropological research points to our ancestors submerging foods in streams and lakes to keep them cold. Refrigeration is a preservation process that works by reducing the activity of enzymes and bacteria.

Preservation techniques make foods more stable and less inclined to grow bacteria and mold. For instance, pasteurization (heating) of milk kills microorganisms which can, in some cases, cause acute illness and even death.

Even with preserved foods you can apply the principle of Wholeness. Look for the food that was preserved with the least amount of adulteration and the greatest amount of nutrient preservation.

The most common preservation methods are drying, freezing and canning. Let's take a look ….

Dry It, You'll Like It

Drying is an ancient and reliable way of preserving foods. If done correctly, it preserves most of the vitamins, minerals and micro-nutrients.

Drying simply involves the removal of water. Without water, the process of decay is suspended. Dried foods can last for years if they are protected against molds, bacteria, worms and other critters. Home dehydrators are commercially available and many retailers sell dried foods.

There are four things to avoid if you want your dried food to be healthy: high temperatures, preservatives (sulfites are the most common), added sugars and salt.

Drying destroys fewer nutrients if done between 95° F and 105° F. Temperatures higher than 110° F greatly increase the rate of nutrient destruction.

A dried food that is kept in a sealed container will last years without the need for preservatives. Sealing reduces exposure to oxygen which triggers oxidation and the release of free radicals (see Chapter 19). The main reason for preservatives is to maintain color. A dried apricot, for instance, will turn brown if preservatives are not used, but it is still full of nutrients. Sulfites, incidentally, are a common allergen and can be deadly for some asthmatics. Most commercially available dried fruits are treated with sulfites and many have added sugar or salt, so read the label carefully.

We tend to think only of dried fruit, but vegetables can also be dried. Because of the popularity of camping, dried vegetables have become more available. They are usually chopped very small or shredded for faster drying. Just as with fruits, avoid preservatives, sugar and salt.

Except for those with pasta machines, most of us buy pasta in its dried form. Beans are widely available in dried form.

The last ten years has seen an explosion of "just add water and heat" foods. Some of these are of quite good quality. The problem is usually the addition of preservatives, artificial flavorings and colorings and hydrogenated oils. Avoid these by reading the labels carefully. You can create your own instant foods by buying organic dried vegetables which are available in most health food and even many specialty grocery stores and mixing them with pasta, a protein source and, if available, fresh vegetables. It's just a matter of adding water to the desired consistency and heating.

Home dehydrators are a great addition to your kitchen, especially if you're a home gardener. Dried foods also make the perfect ration for camping and emergency situations like earthquakes, tornados, floods and "I'm too tired to go to the grocery store" evenings.

The classic book **Dry it, You'll Like It** by Gen MacManiman is the first book on natural dehydration and has been published since 1972. It is filled with delightful recipes for dried crackers, "leathers", and other healthy ways to dry food.

Deep-Frozen Freshness

Freezing is a traditional and healthy way of preserving foods. You can freeze anything from wild blackberries to extra lasagna.

Organic frozen fruits and vegetables are available in some chain stores. As with any packaged food, always read the label. There is no reason for a frozen food to have anything added to the main ingredients. The package should read "Peas" not "Peas, dextrose (a sugar), hydrogenated vegetable oil, green coloring, salt, BHT (a preservative)." The same applies to other frozen foods. You don't need any extras because freezing is the preservation.

A bag of frozen green beans can be cooked in minutes. All you need is a stove, saucepan and whatever spices you like. Frozen foods are easy to use when you can't make it to the farmers' market.

Freezing tips

- If the food is bigger than a cherry or green bean, cut it into smaller pieces. For instance, cherries can be frozen whole (with or without the pit), but an apple will need to be sliced.
- Spread the food out on a tray and place in freezer for an hour or two. This keeps the food from clumping.
- Remove the individually frozen pieces and place in an airtight container such as a self-sealing plastic bag, or glass container.
- Label with the date and place the container in the freezer with the thought you'll be enjoying this food in the future.
- Leftovers such as soups, stews, and lasagna can be placed in air-tight containers in meal-size portions.
- By freezing meal-sized portions and thawing on a rotation basis, you add Variety to your meals.

As with all forms of preservation, nutritional content is decreased when going from fresh to frozen. This is especially true of commercially frozen vegetables and fruits. These are blanched in hot water before freezing. Blanching destroys up to one-third of the vitamin C in vegetables. However, it also kills enzymes that increase decay.

Freshness and wholeness also affect the nutrient content. Therefore, the best frozen foods are the organic ones you pick or buy fresh and freeze at home without blanching.

Can the Cans

Commercial Canning

As a general rule, commercial canning is not a healthy way to preserve foods. There are several reasons for this:

- Poor quality control of the raw fruit or vegetable being canned is one big drawback. When foods are harvested, sorted, washed, cut and packed in large quantities, it's difficult to control for quality. In canning, most people don't notice the inferior quality because it has been cooked. It's more difficult to disguise poor-quality fresh and frozen foods.

- Food value is lost due to high temperatures involved in the canning process. For example, protein and vitamins C and B6 are all reduced by high temperatures.

- Contamination by the metal or plastic lining of the can is dangerous to your health. Plastic can linings are becoming popular because people are worried about the leakage of metal into the food. But danger applies to plastic linings as well. Plastics in foods, especially from soft plastic bottles, are a growing health problem associated with hormonal imbalances and cancer. Some fruits and vegetables are canned in glass jars which are far superior to metal cans, but still require high heat.

- Salt, sugar, colors, and artificial flavors are unhealthy additives you should avoid. Most commercial brands contain these.

Home Canning

For those of you who still home can (I put up a few jars of Italian prunes every year to use as a winter dessert), you bypass three of the above problems - poor quality control, additives, and metal or plastic contamination. In addition, the temperatures used are generally lower.

Home canning is not as nutritious as freezing or drying, but is better than store-bought canned foods.

Freshness Summary

An important part of Wholeness is eating foods that are fresh.

- Try to use foods grown close to home and from your own garden.
- Find a local farmers' market.
- Shop often where you know the produce delivery schedule.
- Eat foods that are in season.
- If fresh foods are not available, dried, frozen and home-canned foods can be used if you pay attention to buying quality products that are organic and free of additives.
- I do not recommend eating commercially canned foods, but life is full of compromises. Your goal is to eat delicious, nutritious foods. Try to buy organic foods in glass containers.

Wholeness Principle Two –

The Organic Orgasm

The second principle of Wholeness is Organic. I'm convinced that buying and eating organic food is one of the most important health and environmental actions you can take.

Farming's field of nightmares

Picture for a minute your last trip through farming country. Or, perhaps you've seen a modern farm in a movie or on TV. *Field of Dreams* showed vast acres of corn disappearing into the sunrise and sunset. It's quite spectacular. In reality, the farmer played by Kevin Costner would have been far too busy spraying pesticides to build a baseball field.

What happens to that field of corn? After growing for weeks with the help of artificial fertilizers and pesticides, it is trucked to the modern ranch. Far more corn goes to feed animals than to feed humans.

The modern ranch is not the vast grassland of John Wayne westerns. It's a series of fences and pens. Seeing hundreds of cows fenced into a grassless pen is not very pretty. Just outside the pens is a line of trucks, burning gas, and are there to deliver the corn from the field of dreams. Gallons of gas are burned for each pound of food. You might say one type of fuel – oil – is being exchanged for another – protein.

Cows in the modern ranch eat non-organic corn and concentrate pesticides and hormones in their fat. Sick from pesticides and not eating their native diet of grass, the cows are given antibiotics. Later the animals are slaughtered and the pesticide, hormone, and antibiotic-laden meat is sent to market. Will you buy it?

On the other hand, if you've ever visited an organic farm you've seen something quite different: perhaps a small field of corn surrounded by fruit or nut trees. Next to that, maybe a field with alternating rows of tomatoes and basil. Chickens or pigs might be getting fat by clearing a field to be used next year for a new crop.

> *"The organic farm is smaller, more intimate and yet more diverse. The plants and animals live more synergistically."*

The organic farm is smaller, more intimate and yet more diverse. The plants and animals live more synergistically. The composted soil has higher amounts of nutrients. Natural fertilizers do what they've done for millions of years; nourish the soil and make artificial fertilizers unnecessary. Pesticides are also not necessary because the soil and plants are healthier. Animals that eat their native diet of grasses and organic foods are less likely to become sick and require antibiotics.

In addition, the organic farm produces more food per acre and is more economically viable than the agribusiness farm, despite what the chemical industry claims. Large agribusiness has one thing going for it, an economy of scale: large amounts of poor quality goods.

Organic gardening takes the place of traditional hunting and gathering. There are too many people and the natural world has changed too much for us to go back to living off the wild. The best we can do is to try and recreate a world in which we have access to fresh, organic foods. The organic farm is an attempt to create a concentrated version of the hunter-gatherer's world. It is not perfect, but it provides us with food that is more nutrient-rich and toxin-poor than what is raised by giant agribusiness.

The organic advantage for you

There has been much controversy, confusion and obfuscation regarding organic foods. Let's walk through the major advantages of eating organic.

Eight major benefits of organic food on your health:

- Higher nutrient content
- Better quality of fats
- No poisonous chemicals
- No preservatives and additives
- No antibiotics
- No synthetic hormones
- No genetic modification
- No irradiation

The Nutrient value of organic foods

In studies comparing the nutritional content of foods, organic foods show higher levels of vitamins and minerals than non-organic.

These higher levels of vitamins and minerals make sense if you consider that non-organic food is grown on soil that is only receiving potassium, nitrogen and phosphorus as the ingredients in artificial fertilizers. These are only a fraction of the nutrients that plants need to be healthy.

A study reported in the *Journal of Applied Nutrition* compared the nutrients of 38 organic to non-organic fruits and vegetables. The nutrients tested included calcium, chromium, iodine, iron, magnesium, potassium, zinc and selenium. The organic foods contained an amazing 200 percent higher nutrient level than the non-organic. In addition, the organic foods were found to have much lower levels of the toxic metals lead, aluminum and mercury.

Studies have also shown organic eggs, dairy and meat to be superior in quality to non-organic. Organic meat, poultry, eggs and dairy products have more carotenes and vitamin E. The vitamin E delays rancidity. The qualities of fats in organic foods are also much healthier for us. Animals that are allowed to roam and freely eat their traditional diet –

known as "free range" eating – contain a better ratio of essential fatty acids. Just like with humans, animals are what they eat.

The United States Department of Agriculture (USDA) which is not exactly a radical organization has published tables showing the decline in vitamins and minerals in non-organic fruits and vegetables that has occurred over the past few decades. Nutrient content has fallen by as much as fifty percent over the last fifty years. Unfortunately, most people are not aware that they're eating more calories and fewer nutrients. Is it surprising that so many people are always hungry?

Artificial fertilizers are the plant equivalent of "enriching" white bread. In the case of bread, over twenty vitamins and minerals are processed out of the wheat, then thiamine, iron and a couple of other nutrients are replaced and the bread is called "enriched." This is retail smoke and mirrors designed to fool the public into thinking they're getting a better product, when they're really being ripped off.

> *"Unfortunately, most people are not aware that they're eating more calories and fewer nutrients. Is it surprising that so many people are always hungry?"*

In agriculture, organic farming supplies dozens of nutrients to the soil, while artificial fertilizers only supply three. Both white bread and non-organic farming are the equivalent of someone holding you up and taking your wallet with hundreds dollars in it, but leaving you with the change in your pocket and calling themselves generous. "Enriched" food and artificial fertilizers are frauds, both to your pocket book and your health.

The advantage of artificial fertilizer is that it is able to force the growth of crops in depleted soil. So, yes, the food is edible and filling, but lacking in nutritional substance. It's a clear example of quantity over quality.

Non-organic = bad fats

When it comes to fat in the diet, quality matters more than quantity. Studies on ingesting high amounts of good-quality natural fats show no negative health consequences. In fact, health usually improves when a person eats a lot of high-quality fat. (For more insight see Chapter 9, Fats 101.)

Much of the negative association between cows and "bad" fat is not the fault of the poor cow. It's because of the way the cow was raised.

Feedlot cows:
- Are fed grains, an unnatural food for cows, resulting in poor health.
- Are loaded with 4 to 6 times more fat than grass-fed cows.
- Contain twice as much saturated fat as free-range cows.
- Are higher in unhealthy omega-6 fats and lower in healthy omega-3 fats when compared to grass-fed.

Grass-fed beef:
- Grass is the natural food of the cow; therefore they become sick less often.
- Contains 2 to 6 times more omega-3 fats. It is the omega-3 fat that is associated with reduced rates of cancer, heart disease, diabetes, arthritis and many other inflammatory diseases. Each day a cow spends in the feedlot its omega-3 level goes down.
- Conjugated linoleic acid (CLA) is 500 percent higher in grass-fed beef and milk. CLA is a type of fat which protects the body from cancer, obesity, diabetes and immune system disorders. The highest known source of CLA is from grass-fed meat and dairy products.
- I'm mainly using beef as an example, but the same applies to free-range chickens, eggs, milk, pigs, turkeys, etcetera.

Based on these facts, it would seem that "Grain fed beef" should not be, as the beef industry would have us believe, a recommendation, but a condemnation.

As with beef, industrially-raised chicken and turkey meat also has abnormal and unhealthy fat levels. Free-range chicken has 21 percent less fat, 30 percent less saturated fat and 28 percent fewer calories. The breasts of free-range chickens are so low in fat they could be classified as "fat free." Free-range chicken also has 50 percent more vitamin A and 100 percent more omega-3 fats.

Free-range chicken eggs have 10 percent less fat, 34 percent less cholesterol, 40 percent more vitamin A and 20 times more omega-3 oils. This gives them the ideal ratio of equal parts omega-3 and omega-6 oils. Recent research and the historic human record show this is the healthiest ratio. On the other hand, factory-raised eggs have an unhealthy 20:1 omega-6 to -3 ratio.

The Paleolithic diet was low in saturated fat and high in omega-3 oils. This dietary pattern was maintained for nearly two million years and only changed recently. This shift away from healthy fat levels came about because of the factory system of farming, cattle raising, and mass dairy production. The farther we've moved away from eating organic, the unhealthier we've become.

Poison, poison everywhere: The sickening consequences of non-organic foods

Besides cheating you of vitamins, minerals and healthy fats, non-organic farming contributes to human and animal poisoning, environmental destruction, loss of topsoil and lowered water tables.

Modern farming practices, from artificial fertilizers to the mass application of pesticides, and genetic manipulation of plants, are seeding wide-spread human and environmental disasters.

Poisoning yourself

Every time you eat a non-organic food you are poisoning yourself. That is a blunt, but truthful statement. If you're not eating organic, you're eating pesticides, herbicides, fungicides, antibiotics and artificial hormones. Some of us are feeding these poisons to our lovers, spouses and children.

Am I exaggerating? The National Academy of Sciences National Research Council found that eating fruits and vegetables may be dangerous for some children because of the pesticide residues. The committee estimated that for some children, total pesticide exposure may exceed the safe dose. They further estimated that exposure could be sufficiently high enough to produce symptoms of acute poisoning in some children. Their study looked for acute or high-level poisoning. The effect of small-dose, long-term exposure was not studied.

The University of Washington found that children consuming non-organic vegetables, fruit and fruit juices had approximately six times the levels of pesticides in their bodies as children eating organic produce.

In the agricultural industry, testing for the safety of pesticides is not based primarily on health considerations, but is conducted by the manufacturers and is designed to monitor "normal" agricultural use. Normal, of course, means whatever the chemical industry can get away with.

In the U.S., a chemical must be proven harmful in order to be taken off the market. European countries, on the other hand, are more often adapting the standard that chemicals must be proven safe before they can be unleashed on the public and the environment.

You can close your eyes and trust the Food and Drug Administration and the Environmental Protection Agency and every other government agency that is supposed to be watching out for your health, but, the fact of the matter is that when you crunch into non-organic breakfast cereal, you are poisoning yourself. If you add non-organic strawberries to your cereal, you've just increased the poison level by another huge percentage.

All government agencies and research institutes will agree that the chemicals used in agribusiness are potentially harmful. What they disagree on is what levels cause harm.

Two and a half million tons of pesticides are used worldwide. Less than 0.1 percent reaches the target pest. The other 99.9 percent is released into the environment where it persists for years, even decades, capable of poisoning you either directly or through the food chain. Of the 50,000 registered pesticides, most were approved for use before the EPA required safety testing.

> *"Pesticides of every category have been found in the groundwater throughout the U.S., in farmland because of crop spraying, and in urban creeks due to home pesticide use."*

The Environmental Working Group (www.ewg.org), a nonprofit research and advocacy organization, estimates that the recommended lifetime exposure limit of some pesticides is accumulating in some humans by the age of five years old.

Pesticides of every category have been found in the groundwater throughout the U.S., in farmland because of crop spraying, and in urban creeks due to home pesticide use. In the Yakima River of Washington State, for instance, researchers found DDT in 100 percent of the fish sampled even though it has been banned for over 25 years. DDT is not degraded in nature so it will be with us forever.

Pesticides are carried around the globe on wind currents. High levels are concentrated in breast milk. This is true even in remote areas with women subsisting on traditional diets. DDT residues are found in 93 to 100 percent of breast milk samples from around the world. Most contaminated breast milk samples have a combination of several pesticides and their breakdown products. So far, all studies have demonstrated that levels of pesticides in breast milk exceed the World Health Organization acceptable daily intake limits.

This is what we've come to - breast feeding is harmful to children! What a world we've created.

Chlorinated pesticides residues (DDT, DDE, DDD, aldrin, dieldrin, heptachlor, heptachlor epoxide and PCBs) have been found in fat samples from women in most European countries, Israel, Tanzania, North and South America. In fact, wherever pesticides are sought, they're found. Eighty-two percent of U.S. human urine samples tested contained pesticides.

A 2003 study by the Center for Disease Control (CDC) found 27 farm and industrial chemicals in every human tested. The Environmental Working Group tested individuals for 210 industrial chemicals and found 167. These are synthetic, new-to-nature chemicals that your body did not evolve to detoxify efficiently.

One last scary thought; these chemicals are not found in nature so our detoxifying systems can't handle them effectively. When your liver can't neutralize a poison your body often sequesters it in a fat cell – thus becoming like a little landmine for later release.

Pesticides: Time bombs in your food

During WWII, DDT was used to control typhus, malaria and lice. Organophosphate (OP) pesticides were used as nerve gas. Sarin, the gas used to kill commuters in the Tokyo subway attack a few years ago, is an OP pesticide.

Organophosphate pesticides are also used to spray houses and apartments for pests and have been linked to birth defects, seizures and neurological disorders in children.

The negative effects of pesticides on humans are not

surprising. They were developed to kill insects by going after their nervous systems. They over-stimulate the nerves causing uncontrolled discharge and even death.

Symptoms of acute toxicity include headache, nausea, vomiting, abdominal cramps, diarrhea, irritability, confusion, convulsions, respiratory depression, blurred vision, muscle twitching, disrupted heart rhythm, anemia and death.

Farm and factory workers with chronic exposure are shown to have poor memories, altered emotional states, fatigue, loss of muscle strength, and slower response time to standard testing. Exposure can also lead to allergies, cancer, and decreased immune system function.

Pesticides have also been associated with chronic fatigue syndrome, infertility and other hormonally related problems.

Chronic Pesticide effects:

Apologists for the chemical industry will say that while high levels of pesticides are toxic, there is no evidence of long-term chronic exposure causing harm. It is true that not enough studies have been conducted (thanks to the chemical industry lobbying efforts), but some studies have been done and they do not put one's mind at ease.

It is known that pesticides, even in small doses, can trigger cancer, injure the nervous system, damage lung tissue, disrupt reproduction, and cause dysfunction of the hormonal and immune systems. Examples of immune system problems are the inability to fight infections, allergy or autoimmune disease.

All of these health problems have been on the rise for the past 100 years and particularly in the past 50 years. Some researchers feel the reason for this is the rise in toxic exposure.

Most toxic foods: And the winners are...

Pesticides are found on all non-organic foods. The 12 most contaminated foods are **strawberries, bell peppers, cherries, peaches, celery, apples, imported grapes, nectarines, kale, lettuce, carrots and pears**. To download a handy shopper's guide, see www.foodnews.org.

One hundred percent of non-organic meat, eggs and dairy contain pesticides, hormones and antibiotics.

Meats, eggs, and dairy are the most contaminated food items because they are at the top end of the food chain. Your non-organic cow has been consuming and concentrating the pesticides found it its feed as well as being given antibiotics and hormones.

The other reason meats, eggs and dairy are laced with the highest levels of contaminants is because they all contain fat which is where most toxins are concentrated.

Strange harvests from across the border

A growing percentage of the U.S.'s agricultural products come from other countries. This is troublesome for several reasons:

- *Weak environmental laws*

  Every country has different laws governing the use of pesticides. Many have much weaker laws than even the U.S.

- *Lack of enforcement*

  Many countries, especially the poorer countries from which we import most of our food, tend to be much more lax about enforcing environmental laws.

- *NAFTA sabotages your health*

  Because of international trade agreements under NAFTA, the U.S. cannot impose its pesticide laws on other countries.

- ***Use of banned pesticides***

  There is widespread overseas use of pesticides that have been banned in the U.S. A recent news article used Myanmar as an example of how illiterate farmers buy outlawed pesticides openly in local markets, mix them without the benefit of proper instructions or protective equipment and spread them at many times the recommended concentration. Often they mix several pesticides to create their own super-poison.

- ***No border protection***

  If your food is coming in from Mexico or other countries with less stringent chemical controls, then you have virtually no protection. You didn't think there were government inspectors checking those Guatemalan strawberries at the border, did you? Theoretically, border security protects you from illegal drugs and terrorists, but doesn't even attempt to look at food-borne chemicals. Virtually no microscopic or chemical testing is done on imported foods.

You are the guinea pig

Because the pesticide industry is not required to prove their products are safe, you are the test animal. Here we are, fifty plus years after the wide-scale introduction of pesticides into our environment, and the government is just beginning to do studies measuring how much "body burden" we have. That measurement is just the answer to one simple question - how much? It only begins to look into the larger question - what harm?

That question, unfortunately, will probably not be answered in a laboratory, but in hospitals across the country by the victims. Will you be a casualty of an unnecessary and destructive experiment in chemical warfare against pests? We already know the pests are winning, what we have left to find out is how badly we are losing.

Treatment of pesticide exposure

Walter Crinnion, ND, writing in *Alternative Medical Review* in 2000, gives the following recommendations for winning the battle against pesticides:

Avoid further exposure

While you cannot completely eliminate exposure to these deadly chemicals because they are carried in the air and water, you can greatly reduce your exposure by consuming organic foods. **Non-Toxic and Natural** and other books can help reduce your home exposure to chemical poisons.

Reduce pesticide impact

Certain nutrients help protect the body from accumulating poisons. Adequate protein, decreased sugar intake, vitamins A, B1, B6, C, magnesium, selenium, antioxidants, and the omega-3 oils all help protect you from poisons. It is no coincidence that these are exactly the nutrients that are high in the Three Wisdoms diet.

Preservatives and additives

Preservatives are chemicals that are added to foods to prolong their shelf life by reducing chemical or microbial degradation. Common examples are BHA, BHT, sodium nitrites, citric acid and calcium propionate.

Additives are a broad category and include any substance intentionally added to foods. There are approximately 3,000 food additives. Additives are used for many reasons. For instance, preservatives are classed as an additive. Other common additives are silicon dioxide, an anti-caking agent, and disodium guanylate, a flavor enhancer. Sugar and salt are the most common additives and are found in almost every packaged or canned food.

Any agent that makes the food more appealing, such

as the coloring in a non-organic orange peel, is an additive, although not always listed on the label.

The FDA is responsible for regulating the safety of food, including additives. The USDA is charged with watching over meat, poultry, and eggs. Controversy surrounds these organizations. Some believe the FDA and USDA do a great job while others fear the influence of big business on our health. History shows there is a revolving-door in which FDA and USDA administrators retire and go to work for the food industries they once were supposed to be watching.

Over one billion pounds of chemical additives are used in foods each year. The average person consumes about 50 pounds annually.

Most preservatives and additives are unnatural to the body because they are man-made. Your body's detoxification systems have only had 50 to 100 years to adapt to these chemicals. How well is it doing? No one knows for sure. Some animal studies, usually with rats, show some additives to be harmless. Other studies have associated additives with an increased risk for cancer. On the other hand, rats aren't people.

One little example of the harm caused by preservatives is that certain preservatives are believed to interfere with vitamin B6 function. A deficiency of B6 is not a minor problem. It is associated with heart disease, diabetes, pre-menstrual syndrome, carpel tunnel syndrome, kidney stones, asthma and depression.

Truth in Labeling

One frightening thing to consider is that there are over 300 foods that require no labeling of additives. Four common ones are bread, ice cream, ketchup and mayonnaise. Breads have been found to contain 80 unlisted ingredients and this is legal!

No Long-term studies

As with most of your environmental chemical exposures, the long-term safety issues of food additives and preservatives have not been studied. Personally, I prefer that a substance has benignly coexisted in the environment for a few million years before I expose my liver to it. That means avoiding processed foods containing man-made additives. I choose to play it safe. My shopping dollars go for organic, additive-free foods like my ancestors ate.

Preservatives and additives in organic foods

Organic foods are full of natural preservatives, flavoring and coloring agents. For instance, antioxidants such as vitamin E and carotenes protect food from spoiling. Carotenes also add flavors and colors.

In my opinion, a food cannot be considered organic, or whole, if it contains added preservatives and additives.

Antibiotics

Antibiotics are another unhealthy additive common in our food supply. "What," you ask, "antibiotics are not good for me?"

Certainly there is a time and place for antibiotics. They save lives every day. However, there is grave concern about their use by the food industry.

All commercial, non-organic animal farming including chickens, pigs, cows, sheep and even fish are given antibiotics. Any animal that does not live in a healthy

> *"We have been led to believe that grain fed beef is the best."*

environment and does not eat a natural diet will develop more infections than an animal living close to how it evolved in nature. The livestock industry saves money by keeping animals in small, confined spaces, depriving them of a wholesome diet, and feeding them antibiotics to keep them alive. This goes for farm-raised fish, also.

Yes, just as humans living in crowded tenements and eating a poor diet are more susceptible to tuberculosis and other infectious diseases, so are animals. At least the human can escape for a little sunlight and exercise; farm animals are not given that luxury.

We have been led to believe that grain fed beef is the best. But grain is an unnatural food for cows. They are ruminants and lack a critical enzyme for digesting starch. They do best on a grass diet. Grains cause bloating, acidosis, liver abscesses and sudden death syndrome in cows. The feedlot cow industry could not exist without antibiotics, hormones and numerous other medications that keep unhappy, unhealthy, poorly-fed animals alive.

Factory farming's negative impact on cows also applies to fowl. When left to forage, chickens and turkeys will get much of their nutrition from grass, clover and greens. When confined to small cages and fed grains, they require antibiotics to keep them alive. These antibiotics persist in the birds' fat and eggs.

By contrast, grass-fed animals, because they are healthier, have lower levels of harmful E. coli bacteria overall and especially low levels of the lethal strains associated with serious gastrointestinal illness and death. Their healthy lifestyle and diet makes them less likely to need antibiotics.

> *"Contrary to most peoples' benign view of them, antibiotics upset nature's balance."*

Twenty million pounds of antibiotics are fed to livestock each year. Only a small percentage is eliminated from the animals. Ninety to ninety-five percent of the residues are found in meat and dairy products consumed by humans.

Contrary to most peoples' benign view of them, antibiotics upset nature's balance. In 2000, the *American Academy of Microbiology* published a paper examining antibiotic resistance. Antimicrobials are commonly found in sewage, seeping into rivers and ultimately flowing into the oceans. Animals and people ingest these antibiotics in their non-organic foods and water. After ingesting an antibiotic, either intentionally or accidentally, some of the bacteria in your body die, while others survive. Those strong survivors then reproduce. The offspring are known as "super bugs" capable of resisting the next exposure to an antibiotic. These bugs are "antibiotic resistant."

A single surviving bacterium can produce over 16 million offspring within 24 hours. With each new generation, more survive the antibiotics. Bacteria are built for survival. Some of them acquire their resistance by grabbing genetic material from other organisms. Cholera, for example, has acquired resistance to tetracycline by stealing genetic material from E. coli bacteria in the human intestinal tract. Cholera has been killing people for thousands of years. Two hundred years ago it was a fairly common cause of death in cities with poor sanitation. Humans finally learned to control it by cleaning up their water supplies. Since the advent of antibiotics, however, cholera has been evolving into a stronger and more deadly organism.

"The widespread exposure to antibiotics from our food supply is contributing to the rise of antibiotic-resistant infections in livestock and humans."

The widespread exposure to antibiotics from our food supply is contributing to the rise of antibiotic-resistant infections in livestock and humans. Thirty-four percent of salmonella, a potentially deadly bacteria common in chickens, is now resistant to five different antibiotics.

The agriculture industry has not gotten the message that we live in a world of interconnected ecosystems. What we feed to our animals is eventually fed to us.

Abigail Salyers, president of the American Academy of Microbiology has stated, "We should start treating antibiotics as an ecological environmental problem."

(Environmental News Network)

Antibiotics kill

The tragic irony of the overuse of antibiotics in the U.S. food supply is that you and I are increasingly likely to die of food poisoning. About 25 people in the U.S. die every day because of food-borne illness.

Antibiotic-resistant infections first appeared in the 1940s, just a few years after the start of the widespread use of antibiotics. They are now one of the major challenges of medical science. The World Health Organization is concerned that there may be a world-wide epidemic of the new resistant strains of tuberculosis - an infection once thought to be almost extinct.

At the same time that this over-reliance on antibiotics is taking place in humans, the meat and dairy industries have had little oversight. The number of inspectors and the amount of testing is limited by budget cuts and little respect for public health measures. In Europe, antibiotics in livestock have been restricted, while in the U.S., lobbyists have pressured Congress to prevent any limits on antibiotic use.

Antibiotics kill friendly bacteria

Antibiotics also cause a problem by being detrimental to the natural good, or friendly, bacteria that inhabit the human intestinal tract. Friendly gut bacteria, when left alone, help manufacture vitamins and keep the ecology of the bowel healthy. The antibiotics in meat and dairy (as well as in medicine) can disrupt the delicate balance of flora. This imbalance can then lead to other health problems. For instance, children without normal intestinal bacteria are more susceptible to allergies, skin problems and upper respiratory infections.

"No antibiotics unless necessary," is a scam

Some fast-food chains are advertising that their beef

suppliers do not use antibiotics; "Unless they are necessary."

This is a ploy to fool you into thinking they have your best interest at heart. The fact is that any cow, pig, chicken or other animal raised in an overcrowded environment and fed an unnatural diet will become sick and require antibiotics. The food industry, by its' very nature, makes the use of antibiotics a necessity.

Whose hormone is that?

Most non-organic cattle are given growth-enhancing hormones. It's an economic reality in the agricultural industry. Ranchers feel they must do this to increase weight and, therefore, profits. Added hormones become deposited in the animal's fat cells. When you eat non-organic meat, you're receiving a dose of synthetic hormones.

Some researchers believe these hormones are responsible for premature sexual development in girls and reproductive problems in males. Girls are developing sexual characteristics at a younger age and male sperm counts are going down.

As with pesticides, additives, and many other chemicals that are now in our food supply, the long-term consequences of synthetic hormone use have yet to be discovered. Are you being affected? What about your children? Or your grandchildren? Evidence suggests all three are affected. No one is spared.

In dairy cattle, the problem is bovine growth hormone (rBGH) which is used for increasing milk production. The USDA allows milk to contain rBGH without a warning label. About 70 percent of U.S. cattle are injected with this hormone. There have been no long-term health studies of rBGH. At least one short-term study has associated rBGH with an increased risk of cancer in humans.

The sick irony here is that this potentially harmful chemical is being used to boost milk production even though there is a milk surplus that results in thousands of gallons being dumped each year.

Most people have enough trouble with their own hormones and, if given a choice, choose to not add milk-enhancing or cow-fattening hormones to their diet.

Genetic modification (GM) of the food supply

As of 2001, more than half of the foods in U.S. supermarkets contained genetically modified ingredients. They have not been proven safe for human consumption (*Scientific American*, April 2001). We have little information on what these altered new species are going to do to our crop land, our agricultural workers, or to ourselves.

Is GM "natural"?

Industry scientists argue that genetic engineering is an extension of evolution and natural selection and is therefore "natural."

This is bad science at its worst. In nature, genes from bacteria do not install themselves in the cells of corn and produce an insecticide. This can only be done in labs by sophisticated laboratory techniques. This type of genetically engineered corn is being planted across America. Our bodies have not evolved to handle this insecticide. And corn has not evolved to know what to do with those bacteria genes.

Plants - at least healthy organic plants - make their own insecticides in small quantities without the help of genes from other organisms. These innate insecticides work quite well, or at least have for thousands of years, when the plant is raised in a natural, mixed-plant environment.

In nature we do not see potato genes mixing with chicken genes nor tomatoes uniting with fish. (Nor pigs and humans mating and creating pigmen.)

GM = stronger insects

Will genetically modifying plants speed up the evolution of

stronger insects? It is reasonable to assume that the answer is yes. This has certainly been the case with insecticide spraying. Stronger insecticides have created super bugs. The scary truth is that neither industry nor government agencies are even asking the question.

Scientists who do this kind of work are driven by success and ego and, although they may have good, but naïve, intentions, their souls are owned by the company store. They rush with single-minded ambition toward patenting new genetic strains with barely a thought as to the broader consequences.

GM proteins are foreign to our bodies

GM foods are, frankly, scary. Their proteins are new and therefore foreign to our bodies. What makes the biotechnology industry think humans will not be allergic to them? We are barely into the GM "revolution" and there are already reports of people reacting with severe allergies.

Will GM reduce the need for pesticides?

I'm especially amused by the argument in favor of GM foods that claims that plants which have been bred to produce higher levels of pesticides will be better for us because this will mean less of a need for spraying dangerous pesticides. Aren't these the same people who have been telling us for 75 years, and who still proclaim, that pesticides aren't harmful? How can GM foods protect us from harmful pesticides if pesticides are not harmful? What will be their next "revolution" – a newer technology that will protect us from GM foods?

The faulty theory behind GM

The GM "revolution" is based on a faulty theory, one that isn't supported by good science. It is entirely based on the premise that one gene produces one protein and this is simply not true. GM scientists insert a gene in a plant hoping to produce a protein that is toxic to insects or will make it grow faster and bigger. But we know from the Human Genome Project that there are only 30,000 to 50,000 genes. This is far fewer than the hundreds of thousands of proteins manufactured within the cell.

The natural cell makes a protein and then modifies it to create dozens, sometimes hundreds of different proteins from one gene. What the bioengineering people can't come to terms with, and don't want to admit, is that the one-gene-one-protein theory is wrong.

When they introduce a new gene into a plant, they are potentially creating hundreds of proteins. And not only are they failing to inform the public and oversight agencies of this, they aren't even testing to see what proteins are made from their patented plants. All they care about is that the one protein they wanted is present because that's enough to establish their ownership.

Industry does not appear to be concerned about the "extra" proteins created from their tinkering. It is our concern, because we don't know what these proteins are, how many there are, or what they can do to us.

A partial list of the potentially harmful effects of genetically-altered foods

1. Fresh-looking food may actually be old and devoid of nutrients.
2. Deleted genes may cause side effects such as suppression of the immune system.
3. Your dog or cat may become cross-contaminated with an abnormal protein.
4. Wildlife will become contaminated.
5. Other crops will become cross contaminated. This is already happening around the world.
6. New, toxic compounds will be formed.
7. Nutritional quality will decline as foods are bred for color and looks.
8. New allergens will be produced.
9. Antibiotic-resistant bugs, bacteria, viruses and fungi will surely develop to outsmart the GM food. These new creatures will be more lethal than their predecessors.

Why you aren't being told the truth?

Are you surprised to read of the potential dangers of GM foods? Were you under the impression they are another wonderful biotech marvel? Maybe you think that way because $250 million dollars is being spent on advertising to convince you that genetic modification is safe. Promoting an unproven and potentially dangerous technology is an interesting way for our society to be spending money when we're suffering alarming rates of food-born illness and even thousands of deaths every year due to lack of funding for food inspectors.

Irradiation: Does it light up your life?

Like most new technologies and chemicals, irradiation is hailed as a giant step forward. But for whom? Certainly not for the consumer.

Industry claims that irradiation is good because it kills bacteria and other microorganisms, thus making our food supply safer. After all, millions become sick every year due to food poisoning.

In the rush to make money on this new technology, no long-term studies have been done to prove it's safety. In laboratory animals, irradiated foods have caused kidney, testicular and chromosomal damage as well as tumors. Irradiated rice has been linked to pituitary, thyroid, heart and lung abnormalities. Children fed irradiated wheat have developed chromosomal abnormalities. Irradiation destroys vitamins A, B1, B2, B3, B6, B12, C, K, and E and folic acid.

First of all, the reason our food supply of meat and dairy is so contaminated is because of the way the animals are raised, not because they're deficient in radiation. Natural, grass-fed animals are less likely to have disease-causing levels of bacteria and the bacteria they do contain are not the "super bugs" or antibiotic-resistant strains, created by feeding antibiotics to feedlot cattle.

Secondly, irradiation, while it kills most bacteria, still leaves behind just enough to mutate and become resistant. Yes, irradiation, just like antibiotics, creates super-strains of bacteria. What's next, turning up the dosage until absolutely no nutritional value remains in the irradiated food?

So, contrary to the millions of dollars in propaganda being pumped out, irradiation only produces one positive - profits for the irradiation industry. The downside is the same result as with pesticides, genetic manipulation and antibiotics - stronger bugs and weaker humans.

Because of industry lobbying, foods are not required to be labeled as being irradiated. If you do see an irradiation label, avoid that food. If in doubt, ask.

Taste and see the difference

Besides the health benefits of organic foods, I'd like to promote two additional benefits. You can even see and taste the difference between organic and non-organically raised fruits, vegetables, meat, dairy and eggs.

Non-organic produce generally doesn't have the deep color (except in the cases where the non-organic is dyed, such as with oranges and farm-raised salmon), nor rich taste of organically-raised produce.

The difference in taste and color is the result of the increased density of nutrients in the organic product. Most of us have had the experience of buying a big, juicy, red tomato, only to discover it was all size and no content. Hydroponic and hot-house tomatoes are notorious for attracting the eye, while disappointing the tongue.

In comparison taste tests, organic meat is preferred over non-organic. The fat in organic meat will tend to be yellow instead of white because of its high content of carotenes, a natural yellowish anti-oxidant.

I have a theory that one of the reasons people tend to overeat is because their sense of taste is not being satisfied. For millions of years people ate a Variety of nutrient-rich foods. They ate leaves, flowers, and even newly sprouted buds. These foods produced a wide array of taste sensations - some subtle, some not. That "memory" of tastes has worked its way into our genetics. When these taste sensations are not being fed, we overeat to compensate for its loss.

The list of good things about non-organic foods is rather short. They are often less expensive to buy so they provide a short-term savings that you will later pay for with your health. They are more readily available. And they provide great financial gain for the owners of corporations at the expense of the consumers' health.

Organic food summary

Ten good reasons to buy and eat organically:
1. Higher levels of nutrients.
2. Lower cholesterol & trans-fats
3. Higher omega-3 oils.
4. Fewer poisonous chemicals.
5. Free of preservatives & additives.
6. Do not contain antibiotics.
7. No added hormones.
8. Naturally evolved, not genetically modified.
9. No harmful irradiation.
10. Tastes better

Wholeness Concept Three:

Low-Processing

Processing the life out of us

The third component of a Whole food, along with it being fresh and organic, is that it hasn't been processed to death.

What is processing? It is the changing of food from its natural state – how it grew – to an altered state. Processing is something that happens by degree. It could be argued that washing your lettuce is a form of processing. Generally speaking though, cutting, grinding, cooking, and chemical alteration are what are meant by processing.

Common examples of processing are the cooking of rice to make it more digestible or the peeling and coring of a pineapple to separate out the softer, sweeter portions from the spiny covering.

You might argue that processing food is beneficial because it helps us find the most delicious and digestible parts of a food. And you would be right. Some forms of processing, such as cutting and cooking, help our digestive system extract nutrients from food.

Traditional processing

For millions of years, while human digestive functions were developing, food was eaten with little or no processing. Breaking, cutting, pounding and, later, cooking were the only preliminaries before chewing.

Our digestion evolved to deal with the natural foods in our environment. We evolved teeth, digestive juices, enzymes, and a digestive canal to deal with native foods. These body functions do a wonderful job of breaking down food at just the right speed and to the right size for absorption and utilization.

The original intent of processing was simply to make plants and animal food more digestible and liberate their nutritional value.

Corn is a great example of what processing can do to or for a food. Some varieties of corn can be enjoyed fresh and raw off the stalk. However, if you want corn in the winter you must dry and store it. Dried corn does not have the same succulent appeal as fresh corn, but it stores for long periods of time. Once dried, it is made edible again by processing. The only choices primitive people had were soaking it for a few days, cooking it whole, or grinding and cooking the flour. These methods of processing have been around for tens of thousands of years and some anthropologists believe they contributed to the transition of ancient to modern man.

Benefits of Healthy Processing – Pre-digestion

Healthy food processing is what you might call the "pre-digestion" of a food. The grinding and cooking of a kernel of wheat, for example, helps us pre-digest a rather hard substance.

The same is true for most foods that were traditionally cut, ground, cooked and otherwise processed; our ancestors were making the food easier to digest. Our digestive system still has to work on these foods to completely liberate the vitamins and minerals, but simple processing prematurely kick starts the process.

Industrial Processing – Going too far

The past 100 years of industrial and chemical science has altered the face of food processing. Simple processing is still done, but foods have been taken into new directions - away from enhancing food value and toward reducing and destroying food value.

Modern industrial processing, with its use of

advanced milling and chemical processing, overly pre-digests our food and removes nutrients.

Wheat is no longer the coarse brown food of our ancestors, but a white powdery substance more resembling sugar. In fact, one of the problems with white flour is that it acts almost exactly like pure sugar in our body. The industrial processing of wheat removes much of the protein, fiber, vitamins and minerals and leaves mostly a simple carbohydrate. Instead of the traditional slow liberation of sugar from our digestive system into our blood stream, white flour floods our system with sugar too rapidly. (See Chapter 32, Diabetes and Blood Sugar, for more on the misery of white flour.)

The same misfortune is true of any food that is subjected to industrial sabotage – large numbers of nutrients are lost.

When does food processing become too much? The scientific literature gives us solid guidelines on how much processing is beneficial and how much is harmful. The evidence shows that food that is processed by "primitive" methods such as cutting, pounding, or low-temperature cooking is not deleterious to human nutrition.

> *"Modern industrial processing, with its use of advanced milling and chemical processing, overly pre-digests our food and removes nutrients."*

Yes, cooking may slightly reduce certain vitamins, but if done correctly, the cooking process liberates more nutrients than it destroys.

Modern processing, on the other hand, has been shown to be unhealthy. Excessive processing changes the molecular structure of the original food and removes important nutritional components.

There are three main ways that foods are overly processed.

Grinding

Grinding refers to the grinding of grains. Traditionally grinding was done with stones and human muscle. Later, animals and wind and water power were used to move large stones to crush grains into crude meal or flour.

Industrial grinding involves motors and steel grinders. These produce tremendous pressure and heat, resulting in grains that are more finely ground. The finer the flour, the more like sugar it acts in your body.

Milling

In milling, fiber and germ are removed from the grain after it has been ground.

Fiber is the outer-most coat of grain kernels, also called bran. Rice bran and wheat bran are common examples. Fiber is more than passive bulk. It aids digestion, elimination, and the ecological balance of bacteria in the gut. It also slows the rate of absorption of simple sugars, thus reducing blood sugar spikes and weight gain. Rice bran, for instance, contains antioxidants, vitamins and minerals. Without it people are more susceptible to constipation, hemorrhoids, varicose veins, gallstones, diverticulitis, diabetes, and bowel cancer, to name only a few common problems. Fiber is also known to reduce cholesterol levels by as much as 30 percent.

The germ is also removed during milling. The germ is the nutrient-rich embryo of a grain or seed. It contains vitamin E, the B vitamins, plant oils and other micronutrients.

White flour is the product of about two-dozen steps that remove or destroy the nutrients in whole wheat. In the process, whole kernels are ground very fine and the fiber and germ are milled away. White flour retains starch, but loses 70 to 80 percent of protein and other nutrients.

As a final "cosmetic" touch, wheat flour is bleached to make it white. Residues of benzoyl peroxide, a common bleaching agent, are left in white-food products.

Pressing and Extraction

These terms refer primarily to the processes - both mechanical and chemical - that have been developed to extract oil from grains and seeds. If you pause to think about it, primitive man would not have eaten much corn, safflower or soy oils. It would have been too difficult of a process. Why muck about trying to extract oil from a soy bean when nuts, seeds and olives are richer in oils and give them up much easier?

It has only been in the relatively recent past that these oils, largely through the wonder of modern chemistry, have been efficiently extracted and sold to the masses. They have even been touted as being good for you. But the opposite is more likely to be true.

The over-consumption of non-traditional vegetable oils, and by this I mean ingesting more than you would consume from eating whole corn or grains, has been linked to a number of human diseases. There is a growing body of evidence demonstrating that the consumption of high amounts of these omega-6 oils are associated with cancer, depression, attention deficit disorders, violent behavior and other nervous system ailments. (For more on this, see Chapter 9, Fats 101.)

The evidence shows that we should stick with the oils that our ancestors ate - what I call "easy press" oils. Easy press oils are those extracted from olives, nuts and seeds. Even coconut oil, after years of unwarranted derision, is now known to be a cholesterol-free healthy oil.

What industrial food processors serve us: Two scary examples

Let's first discuss two foods in their whole forms.

Potato

My favorite example, because it has been so maligned, is the potato. In its whole form, it is an oval tuber that is dug from the ground. The only necessary processing is washing. It could, literally, be plucked from the ground, washed and be eaten whole and raw. Some potatoes are actually quite good, even slightly sweet when eaten raw but it depends on the variety and the freshness. With a little processing such as slicing and steaming, potatoes can be made deliciously enjoyable and a great companion to other vegetables. This natural food contains a variety of nutrients including complex carbohydrate, protein, fiber, potassium, magnesium, vitamin C, folic acid, and traces of many other essential nutrients.

Corn

Fresh corn on the cob is another good example of a whole food. Certain varieties of corn can be picked, peeled and munched raw with delight. The key to this is the freshness. If picked, thrown on a truck, transported several hours, and moved into a grocery store where it has to wait several hours or even days before being purchased and then maybe not eaten until another day or two later, the corn will need to be cooked, buttered, and salted before being eaten. This home processing is a futile attempt to restore the corn's original fresh flavor.

Fresh corn is rich in protein, fiber, folic acid, vitamin C, magnesium, and potassium with traces of many other important nutrients.

Chipping away at health –

How potatoes and corn are processed

Potatoes and corn are two foods that are, unfortunately, not often eaten in their whole, natural forms. In the U.S., a person is more likely to eat potato or corn chips.

These industrially-processed forms have been dried and ground with seasonings, flavorings and preservatives added, cooked and packaged into forms that do not resemble their original whole forms in looks or nutrient value. They have been turned from fresh, whole, nutrient-rich foods to snacks that steal nutrients from your body. The loss of vitamins and minerals that occurs during the processing means that those nutrients will be stolen from your tissues. They are usually cooked with poor-quality oils that trigger oxidation reactions which increases the need for anti-oxidants.

Potato and corn chips are examples of how far modern food technology has moved away from simple food preparation and preservation. Where industrial technology is concerned, it's difficult to find an example that hasn't degraded the quality of food and, therefore, everyone that eats them.

How to choose a healthy processed food

A good orientation to finding minimally-processed foods is to seek out foods that look, smell and taste like they did when they were in their natural growing condition. Examples are a pear off the tree, a sprig of parsley or a grain of raw rice.

The pear and parsley you can eat raw. The rice you must do something to. The key is to do the least. Sprouting and cooking are minimal interventions.

Obviously this approach of eating only foods that look like they did when they were growing eliminates most packaged foods. It's an approach that will greatly increase your intake of nutrients, but it is too purist for most modern people.

The cruel fact is that most packaged products out there are only masquerading as food, but truly have little or no nutritional value. These you should avoid.

On the other hand, there are packaged foods that are of excellent quality. Just like you squeeze an avocado before buying it, you must "squeeze" packaged foods by reading the label.

What do you look for on the label? Search for words that look like foods, not chemicals, as well as whole forms of the food. But remember, the product can be labeled "whole wheat" even if it is mostly bleached white flour. Ingredients are, by law, always listed starting with the food that is the most abundant and proceeding to the least abundant.

Common examples of packaged foods

Pasta/Noodles

Entering your favorite grocery store, you will have many different choices of pasta or noodles. Pasta and noodles are generally purchased dried.

The first products to avoid are the canned ones. They've been subjected to extremely high heat and most of the time will have salt, sugar and other undesirable ingredients added.

Now walk to the dry-food section of your store. There may be dozens of noodles to choose from. Start reading labels. The first thing to look for is what the noodles are made of. Wheat and rice are the most common. Other grains such as spelt, quinoa and amaranth are available in specialty stores and are good choices for adding Variety to your diet.

Earlier I stated the ideal was to eat foods that look like they did in nature. A noodle doesn't resemble a kernel of rice or wheat. On the other hand, noodles have a tradition behind them. They've been around for thousands of years. What would your ancestors have made noodles from? Well, not highly refined, bleached white flour. It didn't exist. They would have used a finely ground whole grain flour. Find the packages made from all or mostly whole grains.

After that, your job is simple. The label on a package of noodles should be quite short. Noodles are only flour that has been mixed with water, rolled out, cut and dried. Sometimes they will have dried vegetables added, which is good, but anything else is unnecessary. They don't need preservatives if placed in an airtight container when you get home.

Breads

Bread, like pasta, has been around for thousands of years. But, what kind of bread? Traditional breads were dark, heavy and hardy − full of fiber and containing most of the components of whole wheat. They required chewing. Besides whole wheat they often contained other whole grains such as rye and barley as well as sprouted grains, nuts and seeds. These breads made up a real meal that traveled well. In fact, they are still one of the gourmet treats of traveling in Europe, especially right out of the brick oven.

White flour breads were rare until the refining process was widely industrialized around 1900. This means that for the past one hundred years the breads commonly available have had most of the nutrients and fiber removed. Bread has largely become a fluff of carbohydrate that, due to chemical preservatives, never goes bad. Most children have never eaten anything other than white bread which is just empty calories. It's no wonder that obesity is an epidemic.

Beans and peas

Traditionally, beans and peas were eaten raw, or dried and cooked later. Surplus beans and peas were dried and stored. Dried legumes were cooked under low heat because that's all that was available. They were not canned under extremely high heat, much less packed with sugar, salt, hydrogenated oils and other refinements of modern living.

Bump and Grind: The mess we've made

In the past few hundred years, and especially in the past one hundred years, the food industry has wreaked havoc on human health by introducing three food-processing techniques - grinding, milling and extraction. Because of these processes, researchers estimate that millions of people suffer unnecessary disease and early death.

The results of the evil three

Eating whole grains is known to improve diabetes control (See Chapter 32), lower cholesterol, and decrease the incidence of heart disease and stroke. Their intake is even associated with reducing the incidence of cancer. The opposite is true of refined grains.

> According to Dr. David Jacobs Jr., of the University of Minnesota, the premature death rate is 15 to 25 percent lower in people who regularly eat whole grains compared with those who consume mostly refined grains. It only takes one serving a day of a whole grain to statistically reduce your risk of death. However, most Americans don't even eat one serving of whole grains daily and only seven percent eat the recommended three daily servings.

It is well established, although largely ignored, that these three processes - grinding, milling and extraction - are strong contributors to most of the chronic degenerative diseases of our time. And besides making us sick, they account for billions of dollars in healthcare costs. Just as government efforts to reduce smoking have saved lives and money, curtailing these types of food-processing would have a profound impact on human health.

What about New and Improved foods?

Any product that is labeled "New" or "Improved" is almost always a food that has been degraded in quality. If the label says "Fortified", then you can be sure that for every nutrient added, several have been removed.

Packaging is also a clue. Be on the lookout for excessive packaging. A potato from the produce section looks like a potato and has not been refined, adulterated or improved. A packaged potato will be a processed potato product and thus requires you to scrutinize the label. These products have often been so cooked and deranged that most of their original nutrients have been lost and whatever has been added, usually salt, fat and preservatives, makes them a meal that steals nutrients.

As if the processed food wasn't bad enough, the materials used in packaging have been associated with genetic defects (*Current Biology*, March 2003).

This process of destruction of nutrients though over-processing is also evidenced in supposedly good or "health foods." Many soy products, for instance, are highly processed and over-packaged. Taking a bean and making it look like beef, sausage or turkey is a feat of industrial manipulation, not sound nutrition.

I'm also skeptical of processing that supposedly makes the food healthier. Probably the first food to be processed in order to "improve" it was milk. Low-fat milk became popular in the 1960's and '70s along with the medical establishment's low-fat, high-carbohydrate diet prescription. The dogma of reducing fat and increasing carbohydrates in the diet has been an overwhelming nutritional disaster. The low-fat craze is part of the reason we are now witnessing an epidemic of obesity. Yet, this misguided strategy is still being clung to. Milk and other foods generally don't need improving. Our ancestors nourished our genes on foods that were fresh, whole and organic – not "improved."

Not so Enriched

"Enrichment" is nutritional and retail fraud. It claims the food has been improved, yet quite the opposite is the case. "Enrichment" replaces iron, thiamin, riboflavin, niacin and, sometimes, calcium. On the other hand, before "enrichment," the food was stripped of several B vitamins, vitamin E, chromium, magnesium, manganese, copper, zinc, fiber and protein. The net effect is a product that should be labeled "degraded."

White "enriched" flour is what most bread, pastas, baked goods, pastries, pizza crusts and breakfast cereals are made from today in the USA. These are the foods that most people eat every day. These products (they don't really qualify as foods) steal nutrition and health from your body. People eat this junk because the corporations selling them spend billions in advertising and misrepresent their products as being healthy because they are "enriched."

Enrichment is a health and retail fraud which is being supported by the FDA, USDA and other government agencies as well as by MDs, the American Diabetic Association, American Heart Association and almost every other mainstream medical society, organization, institution and university. Yes, our taxes are being spent to promote these products. The best these institutions usually do is pay lip-service to eating "complex carbohydrates," a term most consumers either do not understand or take to mean "bread" when it actually should include a variety of whole grains, beans and vegetables.

The enrichment problem also applies to infant formulas in which real food is degraded and sugar added. The result is a high-sugar, low-nutrient feeding that does little more than provide calories and gets the child hooked on sweets. When vitamins and minerals are added to infant formulas, they are often synthetic and out of balance. Manganese has been found in infant formulas at anywhere from three to one hundred times the level naturally found in mother's milk. High manganese is associated with learning disabilities, sleep disturbances, irritability, anorexia, muscle cramps, clumsiness and the commission of violent crimes.

"New and improved," should generally be viewed as you would a skull and crossbones – with terror.

To Cook or Not:
Fire is Nice - in Moderation

Cooking has been with humans for a long time. We've been doing it for at least 40,000 years. Some anthropologists see evidence for cooking dating back 250,000 years.

Cooking enabled early humans to consume a broader range of foods by making them more digestible. Cooking, some researchers propose, helped Homo sapiens thrive. Anthropologic evidence suggests that cooking foods did not start a decline in human health, but was part of an evolutionary fork that separated us from other primates.

It has even been argued that cooking was an integral part of the civilizing of mankind. The domestication of grains was a major civilizing influence and grains were, for the most part, cooked before eating.

Cooking also kills unwanted bacteria.

Primitive humans would have been cooking whole foods at low temperatures. Before the advent of pottery vessels, food was cooked primarily by roasting over an open fire or pit roasting. You might be familiar with the method of wrapping a food in banana leaves, burying it in sand, building a fire on the surface and waiting several hours for dinner to be served. It was the original crock pot. With the advent of vessels, food was parboiled, steamed or baked in baskets, low-fire clay vessels or clay ovens which are all relatively low-heat

> "Cooking helps break down or predigest a food. If done over low heat, most of the nutrients are preserved. The higher the temperature, the more nutrients are lost."

methods of cooking.

Cooking helps break down or predigest a food. If done over low heat, most of the nutrients are preserved. The higher the temperature, the more nutrients are lost.

Raw food advocates argue that cooking destroys important enzymes necessary for digesting the food. They claim our digestive juices are adequate for breaking down any food in its raw form and that cooking is bad. I don't see their claim being supported by anthropologists. I have also seen some very sick raw food proponents in my practice.

Raw grains are not practical or palatable to most modern humans except when sprouted. Some vegetables are soft and easily digested while others, such as broccoli, are fibrous and difficult to digest.

Even if humans did once have the digestive enzymes necessary to break down all foods in their raw form, they are likely deficient in these enzymes now. Raw food advocates further argue that there are enough enzymes in the food to "self-digest" itself. This may be true of very fresh, organic foods, but enzymes die quickly. Unless you're eating fresh out of the garden, there are probably few enzymes left in your vegetables. Furthermore, which of our modern foods were eaten by hunter-gatherers? Few to none. Foods have been selected and cultivated over thousands of years for their taste, not their enzyme content. If ancient man ate anything resembling an apple, it was small, hard and tart and more like a crabapple, not a Granny Smith flown in from New Zealand.

There are no known human groups or tribes that exist solely on raw foods. Modern peoples that still follow the hunter-gatherer lifestyle cook their foods, even those living in hot climates.

The cooking of grains is a special case. Grains were not eaten by primitive peoples to any great extent. They only came into significant use about 9,000 years ago, long after fire was introduced. So, pre-agricultural early humans would have consumed only small amounts of wild grains that were probably cooked.

On the other hand, most people in the U.S. eat too many cooked and even over-cooked foods. We tend to overcook fresh vegetables until they are soft and nutrient depleted. We also consume canned foods that have been subjected to very high temperatures. The large-scale experiment in microwave cooking that the world is now experiencing is also nutritionally troublesome.

A recent study in the *Journal of the Science of Food and Agriculture* (October 2003) found that boiling of broccoli led to a 66 percent loss of flavonoids compared to fresh raw broccoli. Pressure cooking lost 53 percent and microwaving lost 97 percent!

The best way to retain the wholeness and freshness of a vegetable is to eat it raw or to lightly steam it. Light steaming has a negligible affect on the nutrient content. This is done by placing the vegetable in a steamer basket with a small amount of water. Ideal cooking times are very short – just a few seconds for green leafy vegetables such as chard, kale and spinach and a minute or two for tougher vegetables such as broccoli, cauliflower and Brussels sprouts.

For green leafy vegetables, after the water has been brought to a boil, remove the pot from the stove, keep the lid on, and let the vegetables steam until slightly soft and bright green. The time will depend on the amount of vegetables in the pot and the size of the vegetable. Cutting vegetables into small pieces decreases the cooking time. By using arm energy - cutting - you save stove energy.

The benchmark is to cook the vegetable only enough to slightly weaken the cell walls. Inside these cells are the vitamins and minerals. Once the wall is weakened, your teeth and digestive juices can do the rest of the work. On the stove-top, this means being able to penetrate the vegetable with a fork, but having the vegetable still be firm enough to support the fork. If it's over-cooked, the fork will enter as if it was butter.

Slow-cooking at low temperature is the way to go. Avoid high-temperature, pressure or microwave cooking.

Processing Summary

A processed food has been broken, burned or disfigured in some way. It has fewer nutrients and is farther way from what humans traditionally ate.

When you're standing in your favorite grocery store with florescent lights blazing, it doesn't take long to separate real food from processed if you ask yourself a few questions.

- Is this a food that is similar to foods that were eaten by hunter-gathers? Or has it been distorted and packaged?

  Granted, even the modern organic apples (and most other fruits) are far different from their pre-agricultural ancestors. A lopsided organic apple (especially if it has a worm hole) is closer to its original form than the gigantic, perfectly proportioned, wax-covered non-organic varieties. In growing, the plant that is most stressed by weather and other environmental factors will contain the higher amount of nutrients so choose the ugly duckling with the heart of gold.

- Is the food time-tested and not lab fabricated?

  If it comes in a box, read the label and look for ingredients that aren't foods. In fact, if it has a label, it automatically falls into the suspicious category. Just like with a legal contract, lots of small print may mean that someone is trying to pull one over on your health. Not that there aren't some good-quality organic packaged foods, but they are the exception. Many "natural" products (such as soy burgers) only vaguely resemble the real article. Buyer beware.

- Has the food been stepped on?

  "Stepped on" is drug-slang for adulterating with foreign substances. Again, read labels and watch for fillers, binders, preservatives, and dyes. If the food has been "fortified", it has probably had a lot of its nutrient-value removed, or didn't have much to begin with. (To adequately fortify a can of soda, you wouldn't just add calcium. You'd start with fiber, then a couple of dozen vitamins, minerals and other food factors, then remove the sugar...)

- Has it had anything removed?

  Did some chemist try to improve upon nature by removing something, like the fat? Was the fiber removed during milling? Stay as close as you can to a Whole food.

It's your choice; eating a food with millions of years of evolutionary biology, and proven nutritional strength, or the product of a chemistry lab.

Whole Foods Summary

I know that at first this concept of wholeness might seem overwhelming. Give it time. In a few weeks it will be second-nature to you. Remember, there are three qualities to a whole food:

- **Fresh**
- **Organic**
- **Low processing**

You can determine if a food is Whole by quickly running through a few questions.

1. Is the food fresh?

How old is it? When was it picked?

These questions don't matter much if you're eating processed and packaged food, but if you're eating natural, whole foods, they are important questions.

The best solution for guaranteeing freshness is to grow it yourself. Next best is to be on friendly terms with your rosy-cheeked produce person. Ask her if the melon is from your state, or flown in from far-away places. Avoid old, long-distance, hard-traveled fruits and vegetables. Buy produce that is in season for your area. You may be forced to try something that's never crossed your taste buds before, but your health will prosper and you'll probably like it. Your new taste sensation will give you something to talk to your friends about.

If you can't find quality fresh produce, look for organic dried or frozen foods. They're becoming more readily available. If you ask, you create a demand. Smart store owners pay attention to demand.

2. Is it Organic?

Was this food grown using organic-farming methods? Is the meat or dairy product organic or grass fed?

If it's organic, it has more vitamins and minerals and contains no residues of chemical poisons, hormones, antibiotics and is not irradiated or genetically modified. Look for the organic label (although the government is trying to water-down organic labeling guidelines). Know your produce person. Don't confuse "low pesticide residue" with "certified organic." You not only want to avoid all chemical contamination, but you want food that has been grown on rich, cared-for land.

Aren't you being bombarded with enough toxic chemicals from the environment? Why pay for food contaminated with pesticides, herbicides, antibiotics and hormones? If you think organic foods are too expensive, ask yourself; what could be more of a waste of money than eating foods full of poisons and without nutrients? Or, simply ask yourself, what do I live on? Your answer may include love, family, friends, spiritual and educational development and good nutrition.

As you stand in your local store inspecting foods, ask if they are going to give or take nutrients from you. Do you want a meal of steel or a meal that steals?

3. Is it overly processed?

You want the whole and nothing but the whole food.

When someone is trying to sell you a new food, the proof of quality is in how close it is to a food that grows in nature. Read the list of ingredients. Watch out for "refined" or "enriched". And no, a potato that is flat and salty and comes in a package is not a whole potato. It's a nutrient-robbing varmint.

Chapter 18

Bringing the Wisdoms together

My sincere hope is that you now see the Three Wisdoms as simple, sound, concepts that you can apply to shopping and eating. Yes, there is a wealth of information here, but once you get it and understand the fundamentals, it will become easy for you to apply. Again remember the mantra – Regularly eat a Variety of Whole foods.

How long will it take to see results?

I'd like you to give **Nutrition-1-2-3** at least a four-week trial. Although some people feel better sooner, my experience is that most people will feel a difference in three to four weeks. I have seen hundreds of my patients apply this program. Many feel better in as short as one week. All of them feel that the program benefits them to some degree. Most find it so rewarding - and so easy - they want to continue.

Obviously, if you are overweight, have diabetes, heart disease or other major health problems, your recovery will take longer. But, most of these people are amazed just how quickly positive dietary changes improve their health. Proper diet makes a difference. Give it a chance.

Does this program apply to my children?

If you have children, you should be even more motivated to learn and apply sound nutrition. **Nutrition-1-2-3** is applicable, even critical, to childhood nutrition. If you can start your child on a healthy program from day one, or even pre-one, while you're pregnant, your child will have a head-start that even teenage dietary indiscretions won't erase. If you start them young, they will develop the consciousness and taste that will keep them eating wisely for the rest of their lives.

Additionally, type 2 diabetes is rising steeply among children. Thirty years ago it was rare to non-existent in kids. Now, thousands have been diagnosed with this debilitating and deadly disease. The U.S. government's Center for Disease Control estimates that one in three children born today will develop diabetes (*Journal of the American Medical Association*, October, 2003). The long term complications of diabetes include heart disease, obesity, cancer, visual impairment, and circulatory insufficiency.

Think about diabetes the next time you take your kids to a Junk-In-A-Box for a "treat." Diabetes is a time-consuming, expensive and deadly disease which is directly linked to eating habits.

Other common childhood conditions, such as chronic ear infections, allergies, attention deficit disorder, and hyperactivity can also be treated successfully through good nutrition. Eating well is beneficial for everyone in your family.

Summary of the Three Wisdoms –
Comparing the Three Wisdoms to the Standard American Diet

Here are some quick comparisons between Three Wisdoms Meals and the Standard American diet (SAD).

Three Wisdoms	SAD
Meals of Steel – make you stronger	Meals that Steal – rob nutrients
Organic	Non-Organic
Whole	Processed
Fresh	Rotting
Regular meals & snacks	Irregular & missed meals
Variety of foods	Repetitive eating
Provides Nutrients	Steals Nutrients
Dense nutrition	Few or no nutrients
Foods look like grown in nature	Boxes/cans/concentrates
Protect you from aging	Contributes to aging

Three Wisdoms	SAD
Protects from chronic disease	Contributes to chronic disease
Less likely to need medicines	Regular medication use
Healthy Children	Unhealthy children
High Energy	Low Energy
Stable Blood Sugar	Hypoglycemia or diabetes
Reduced cancer risk	Increased cancer risk
Clear, healthy skin	Acne, eczema & other skin conditions
Healthy weight	Excess weight

To me, the choice is clear. Your genetic ancestors flourished eating by the Three Wisdoms. Modern scientific research supports their superiority over the standard American diet. I hope you see the Wisdom of **Regularly eating a Variety of Whole foods.**

SECTION IV

Wisdoms in Action - Shopping, cooking and traveling

Chapter 19

To Market, to Market – Three Wisdom Shopping

You're well-intentioned. You want the best nutrition for you and your family. But here you are standing at the entrance of your local grocery store with a sweaty palm clenching your ecologically-friendly shopping bag.

Are you ready to run the food-industry gauntlet? Are you confident you can win against the nutrition robbers? Shopping can be an unfriendly experience unless you're prepared.

Your mantra

Before you grab your shopping bag and yell "Charge!" repeat the mantra, "Regularly eat a Variety of Whole foods," until it becomes second nature. Repeat this mantra (perhaps silently if you want to avoid stares) on entering the store and each time you pick up a food. This mantra will ground you in good nutrition and make it possible for you to skip most of the aisles that are filled with canned and processed foods.

Tips to make you a shopping victor

Your friend the shopping list

A shopping list, especially if you're buying for a family, helps you focus on healthy foods. It's also a time-saver. Why meander up and down aisles when you can go directly where your shopping list leads you?

When shopping for a family, it can be quite helpful to have a reusable list. This is a sheet of paper with all the foods you buy listed by food group. Groups include: Fresh fruit, fresh vegetables, grains, legumes, nuts/seeds, fish and meat, dairy, frozen, spices, and miscellaneous. Leave space after each heading to write in what you need.

Under each heading, you can include a list of the specific foods you rotate through your diet. As an example, under legumes would be: black, pinto, mung, azuki, etc. This helps you remember to rotate your foods for variety. Do the same for the other groups also.

For greater efficiency, you may lay out the list in the order of your favorite grocery store aisles. You can then follow the list around the store picking out what you need.

You only have to make the list once. After that you can copy the original or print it from the computer. The list can be kept on the refrigerator or another convenient place so that when you run out of a food, its name can be circled. Electronic memory machines can also be used. When shopping you can go directly to what you need and not stand there trying to remember. (See Section IX for example)

Choose the battleground

You can improve your chances of victory against disease if you select the field of battle. Many cities have natural food stores that are part of national chains and are becoming common such as Whole Foods, Wild Oats, and Trader Joes. Your city may also have mom-and-pop health food stores or even a food co-op. You still need to be careful to read the labels, but your chances are better at finding organic, whole foods at these stores.

There is a rule of thumb about shopping in stores that advises you to always shop on the periphery, where the fresh foods are usually stocked, rather than in the center of the store where packaged and canned foods are displayed. It's not a hard and fast rule, but it does work as a general guideline. Organizing your shopping this way can also save you time. It's those middle aisles stocked with 32 different kinds of canned soups that can really slow you down – until you realize there's nothing there with much nutrition in it anyway.

Knowing your local produce stand or farmers' market can give you access to fresh, whole foods. If the owner knows there are customers for organic fruits and vegetables, he or she is more likely to seek out a source. Farmers markets commonly carry a wide variety of fruits and vegetables, as well as fish, organic meat, chicken, eggs, and dairy products. They're also a great place to pick up local flowers that haven't been sprayed and flown in from distant lands. If you belong to a subscription-produce service, the organic farmer will deliver the produce to your door weekly, saving you a trip to the mine-field of shopping.

Watch for booby-traps

Be especially wary of any food in a package or can. Become familiar with how to read labels (see Section IX at end of book). Ingredients are listed in order of percentage. Whatever is first on the label will be the most plentiful, and down from there.

A good way to approach a label is to imagine what the foods' basic ingredients are and to make them your benchmark. To make bread, for instance, it only takes flour (preferably 10 percent whole wheat), water and yeast. Anything else on the label is extra. That extra might be a negative addition such as sugar or it might be a positive addition such as sunflower seeds, oats, raisins, and other health-building ingredients. The same strategy applies to everything from the simple – oatmeal only needs oats – to the complicated – lasagna basics include the noodles, tomatoes, cheese and spices.

Speaking of pastas, they are often made from semolina wheat, but you can also find them made from whole wheat, rice, quinoa and amaranth flour. These add variety to your meal planning. And remember, your basic noodle is made from flour and water.

I repeat: generally avoid foods with labels, but if you must eat a packaged food, read the label carefully. At first this will seem tedious, but soon you will recognize the better brands and products. Right now you may have some unhealthy food-buying habits. Acquiring new habits requires a few weeks of applied consciousness.

Shopping Summary

You can be triumphant in the struggle for health if you have a mantra that sends food-processors into a panic. **"Regularly eat a Variety of Whole foods,"** does to them what hearing "IRS audit," does to you. Have a shopping list, preferably in writing. Your shopping-list allows you to get in and out without being wounded by health robbing foods. Picking a health-friendly place such as a health-food store, gives you a better chance of success but don't let your guard down. Always read the labels.

By following these suggestions you can make shopping less lethal and turn it into a more healthy experience.

Chapter 20

Wisdoms in the Kitchen –

Building health one meal
at a time

OK, you're in the kitchen, feeling hungry, maybe even thinking about calling for take-out, but you decide it's about time you started using your kitchen as a place to restore health rather than as a feeding trough.

Starting over

When first getting started on a nutrition program, you may need to follow the old axiom, "Out with the old and in with the new." It's not a waste of money to throw away unhealthy food. The money was already wasted, the land was already poisoned, and gas was already burned bringing it to market. Much harm has already been done so why do more by putting it in your body? THROW IT AWAY. Then get thee to the grocery store armed with your list and mantra - "Regularly eat a Variety of Whole foods."

Fill your kitchen with whole, fresh foods and a healthy attitude. If you have the right ingredients and a few simple utensils you can create a six-course gourmet dinner or a five-minute power meal. Remember, just like learning any new behavior, for the first few weeks it may seem difficult, but eventually you will develop healthy food-preparation habits.

Plan Ahead

If you are going to Regularly eat a Variety of Whole foods, having the right ingredients, the right utensils and enough time are essential. If you have plenty of time, then you will have fewer problems. If your time is limited, then planning is even more important. Fixing meals for others also requires additional planning.

Meal plan

Whether you keep it in your head or write it out in detail, you need a plan. The plan will guide your shopping and cooking. The plan can be an elaborately composed, computer-generated, hard-bound tome or a scribble on your wall calendar. Whatever works for you is the right way.

Since you have a lot of Whole, organic foods in your kitchen from your shopping (right?), the only thing you have to think about in meal preparation is Variety.

Variety

Variety, as you recall, is easily accomplished by dividing foods into Food Groups.

Food Groups

Each meal and snack should contain some carbohydrate (starch), protein and fat. For most people it is easiest to build a meal by starting with the protein requirement. Once you've established the type and amount of protein, then add the starch. Fat often takes care of itself when you're eating organic whole foods.

Protein

Let's say your requirement for protein is 70 grams daily. (See Chapter 8, Protein 101 for how to determine your protein needs.) You want that amount divided up throughout the day so you're controlling the release of energy and maintaining even blood sugar.

Now you divide that 70 grams into Regular feedings throughout the day. For instance, you decided to have 15 to 20 grams of protein at each meal and 5 to 15 at each snack. You now have a pretty good idea of how much protein to have at whatever meal or snack you're preparing. At first, you will want to pay attention to these numbers, but after a little practice - a week or two - you will know how much protein to eat without making calculations. A healthy habit will have developed.

After knowing how much protein you're going to have at a particular meal, then decide what kind of protein. Meat eaters have a wider palate to choose from while vegetarians are more limited in their selections. But whatever your preference, remember Variety.

Add Variety to your protein intake by rotating different protein sources through your meal plan: fish, legumes, nuts, tofu, meat, tempeh, chicken, eggs, etc. And remember to always choose Organic.

The type of protein you decide on will influence the amount of starch and fat you need to add. For instance, if you choose a piece of organic chicken, then you will want some starch also. On the other hand, if your protein is from beans and grains, then you probably don't need to add a starchy food such as potatoes or corn because the beans are already a combination of protein and starch. You can, of course, always add plenty of carbohydrates from green, red and yellow vegetables (chard, spinach, salad greens, asparagus, etc.) because these are high in vitamins and minerals, but low in calories.

Carbohydrates

Starch selection is a little more complicated because so many foods fall into this category. Grains, beans, vegetables and fruits all contain starch.

Emphasizing vegetables is an excellent way to cut calories while supplying vitamins, minerals and antioxidants. Green, red, yellow and orange vegetables are very low in calories. Only potatoes and squash have significant levels of calories.

If you're having grains or starchy vegetables such as potatoes, the amount you need falls dramatically unless you require a high-calorie diet or want to gain weight. In general, vegetables and fruits are your best sources of carbohydrates. They're rich in vitamins, minerals and fiber, while low in calories.

Grains, either cooked alone or made into bread or pasta, are a source of complex carbohydrates, protein, fiber, vitamins and minerals. One of the most common mistakes that people make in their nutrition is relying on bread as a source of carbohydrate. To coin a phrase: Man and woman should not live by wheat alone. Rotating some of the less-commonly eaten starches such as sweet potatoes, millet, squash, barley, parsnips, quinoa, and various beans into your diet enhances your overall nutrient intake and reduces the development of food allergies. Many people find that reducing wheat is a great way to lose weight because wheat has an addictive quality that stimulates appetite. This is caused by the release of mood-elevating endorphins.

If you are a vegetarian you're probably taking in plenty of carbohydrates because all of your protein sources contain carbs. Eat little or no carbohydrate-only foods. Potatoes are a poor choice for a vegetarian because they contain little protein. Millet, quinoa, legumes, nuts and seeds are better choices because they have higher amounts of protein.

Generalizations are difficult in nutrition, but most

people in modern society are not burning enough calories in their daily lives to need much in the way of starchy foods, especially breads and potatoes. I suggest a portion size about the size of your fist for carbohydrates. Those of you doing manual labor or heavy exercise may require more.

Fats

Fats often take care of themselves if you are Regularly eating a Variety of Whole foods. Meats, nuts, seeds, dairy, eggs and certain foods such as avocados have enough fat to cover your needs for a meal.

On the other hand, if you're having a low-fat meal of beans, which provides protein and starch, but little fat, then you will need to add a small amount of fat in the form of nuts, olives or a splash of healthy oil. The classic example of a legume meal with a fat is pork-and-beans. The pork, high in fat, adds the missing ingredient to balance the protein and starch of the beans. Of course, your added fat might be olive oil, or walnuts, or whatever else your imagination and taste buds allow.

A salad with organic chicken strips provides you carbohydrates and protein, but little fat (organic chicken breast is very lean). You will need an additional tablespoon of extra-virgin olive oil, or olives, avocado, nuts or something else with fats.

While I'm not emphasizing fats, that doesn't mean I don't think they're important. They're critical for good health. All societies use the fats that are available to them – from whale blubber to coconut oil. Traditionally-consumed **organic** fats and oils, even butter, have been shown to be healthy in the diet.

Kitchen Equipment

The number and types of utensils you have in your kitchen will depend on how elaborately and how much volume you cook. Here are a few basics:

- Several sauce pans of various sizes with well-fitting lids are essential. I recommend using stainless steel as it spreads the heat better than aluminum. Although not conclusive, there is concern about aluminum cookware increasing blood levels of aluminum and potentially contributing to nerve damage.

- A steamer tray or two that fit inside a saucepan are nice for steaming vegetables, but are not necessary. They are filled with holes that allow the steam from boiling water to cook the food in the steamer. Asian markets are a good place to find these. Otherwise, steam in a saucepan using a small amount of water in the bottom.

- One or two skillets, cast iron or stainless steel, also with lids. Avoid non-stick coatings as they give off unhealthy gases.

- A heat-resistant dish and lid for oven baking.

- A sharp set of knives and a sharpening stone are a must. Respect your fingers!

- Large spoons and a ladle for soups.

- Tongs for grabbing hot food.

- Food processors, blenders and mixers are not necessary but are convenient, especially for preparing large meals. The most important thing to consider when buying electric appliances (besides electric-shock safety) is ease of cleaning. If it's difficult to clean you'll quickly lose interest in using it. The only electrical kitchen appliance that I regularly use is a small grinder. Although they are usually sold for grinding coffee, I use them for grinding dry ingredients such as flaxseed, nuts and spices. These grinders do not have to be washed, only wiped out.

Microwave Caution

A few studies have been performed on the safety of microwave cooking and its effects on nutrition. The results of these studies have not been good. When blood tests were performed on people consuming microwaved food, their nutrient levels were at the "lower limits of normal" compared to subjects eating conventionally cooked foods. During a second month of cooking with a microwave, the test group's blood nutrient levels fell even further. Remember, vitamins are essential nutrients that your body does not manufacture; you must get them from your diet.

A study comparing boiling, steaming and microwaving showed that steaming retained the most nutrients and microwaving the least. Over 80% of nutrients were lost in microwaved foods!

The microwaving of breast milk causes the breakdown in the milk's natural antibiotic activity. Microwaving alters the structure of cells to form compounds not found in nature.

I do not recommend my patients place themselves in harms way with the use of microwave ovens. This is another of those mass experiments which uses humans as guinea pigs.

Eating in the raw - Salads

Perhaps the simplest meal you can prepare is a mixed salad. The great thing about a salad is that they can be an extremely simple snack – literally a variety of chopped greens – or, with just a little more work, a complete meal which includes carbohydrates, protein and fat. Emphasize mixed – as in lots of different stuff in the salad - for Variety.

Carbohydrates for a salad

This list includes lettuce (many types), spinach, radicchio, tomatoes, romaine, frisee, radishes, cucumbers, peppers, arugulas, etc. Colored vegetables are mostly carbohydrates and yet are low in calories.

You can add a few more calories with the addition of steamed and diced potatoes and yams or chop up a leftover baked potato for additional starch. Don't forget sliced or grated carrots, beets or rutabagas. We're talking taste sensations!

Cooked whole grains, pasta and legumes can also be added for more carbohydrates and some protein.

Pear, apple, orange or grapefruit slices and grapes and berries all add a nice "sweet" contrast to the slightly bitter vegetables.

Proteins for a salad

Diced fish, tofu, chicken, ham, turkey, hard-boiled egg, cheese, nuts, garbanzo and other beans all add protein to a salad. Smoked salmon or sardines can also be excellent additions. These can be used either as a light garnish or as a major protein helping, depending on what else you're eating. Leftovers often find a second life when diced into a salad.

Fats for salads

Avocado slices, nuts, seeds, olive oil, nut or seed oils (try walnut oil!) and whole or chopped olives all contain quality oils. Remember that if you've already added nuts, eggs or cheese, you already have some fat in your salad and may just need a light dressing.

Pre-made salads

Some grocery stores are now stocking pre-made salads or

pre-mixed vegetables which save preparation time. They also tend to reduce spoilage. Select the package with a Variety of ingredients and check for the freshest date stamp.

The highest quality salads will be Organic and not contain any sulfite preservatives which are common triggers of asthma and allergies.

Salad dressings

The constant ingredients in most salad dressings are oil and vinegar or lemon. The variables, besides the kind of oil and vinegar, can be anything from a splash of mustard, to egg, to fish sauce. It's best to make your own as most pre-mixed dressings use non-organic ingredients and poor-quality oils such as corn and soy. Good dressing oils are olive, flax, walnut, sesame or other nut and seed oils. A basic proportion is two-thirds oil to one-third vinegar, but this will vary according to your taste and what other ingredients you're adding.

Basic Dressing Recipe

If you have no idea how to make a salad dressing, here's a basic recipe that uses ingredients found in most kitchens or in a store not too far away. This is a basic starter dressing.

Ingredients:
- ½ cup of extra virgin olive oil.
- 2 tablespoons of vinegar (red wine, apple cider or balsamic) or lemon juice.
- 1 clove of minced garlic or ginger

You simply throw all these ingredients together in a jar and shake. Now taste it. Not vinegary enough? Prefer more garlic? You can figure out what to do next.

Do you like your dressing with a little snap? Add mustard. Prefer a tomato dressing? Add a fresh tomato and do the whole thing up in a blender. Other common additions are pepper, orange juice, fresh crushed basil and oregano. Have a discussion with your taste buds. The whole process takes less than ten minutes (quicker than making a trip to the store) and when sealed in a dark container and refrigerated, it will last for weeks.

Cooking foods

Baby Steps: First boil water

This is not a cookbook. Millions have already been written. Most are too complicated for the novice. Before graduating into more elaborate recipes, you must know the basics.

Much of cooking starts with knowing how to boil water. If you can boil water, you can cook healthy meals. After learning to boil water, you can master simple baking.

Cooking rice and other grains

You may have noticed, but most grains are a bit too hard to eat raw. Boiling them is easy.

Basic Boiling

If you're a stickler for absolute measurements, you'll hate me. I don't even use a measuring cup when cooking grains. My method is to pour enough of the grain to cover the bottom of a sauce pan (from ½ to 1" deep). I then pour in enough cold water to cover the grain, plus about ½". I bring the water to a boil and then turn it down to simmer on low. The grain is finished cooking when the water is gone. I know, not exactly Julia Child, but it works for me.

Different grains absorb different amounts of water, so I've included an easy reference chart (See page 239)

Cover the grain and water mixture with a tight-fitting lid. Turn the stove on high and bring to a boil (two to five minutes). As soon as the water begins boiling, immediately reduce the heat to low.

It's best if you do not remove the lid during this process. You can usually hear the boiling. Continue cooking on low heat for ten to thirty minutes. The time difference is due to the size and hardness of the grain as well as the heat of your stove. Rice is bigger than millet. Quinoa is softer than rice, etc.

The best way to figure out if your grain is cooked is to take a peek after about ten to twenty minutes. When the grain is done the water will be gone and there will often be small bubbles formed on the top. You can always slip in a fork and try a bite. It should be soft and chewy but not crunchy. If the water is gone and the grain is not cooked, then add more water and remember for next time. If the grain tastes done, but there is still water, then you added too much. Simply drain off the extra and use it for a soup starter. If you cook the grain too long it will stick to the bottom of the pan (this is considered a delicacy in some countries) and will make clean-up more difficult.

If done right, the grain will tumble from the pan without sticking and washing the pan will take seconds.

Rice cookers are easy to use and will also work with other grains, but most are made with aluminum or coated with plastic. Both of these should be avoided.

If you're going to cook a grain, you might as well cook more than what you need immediately. Leftovers can be reheated or mixed in to other dishes. Salads, steamed vegetables and soups can all be made more nutritious this way. Leftover millet, for instance, can be saved in the refrigerator and reheated in a steamer later.

Gourmet Grain

Once you've mastered basic grain cooking, you are only limited by your imagination. A step toward gourmet is to add herbs and spices during cooking - diced onion, chopped garlic, saffron, or a bay leaf. Any spice that sounds good to you is fine.

You can also throw in other foods and cook them at the same time - slices of peppers, diced carrots, and broccoli. A quick-cooking vegetable like spinach would be added in the last 5 seconds of cooking the grain, while chunks of winter squash would need to cook as long as the rice. Grated vegetables cook faster than whole ones. It's a matter of paying attention to size and density.

Just about any other food can also be added to the pot including eggs (whole or stirred in), nuts, seeds, and even meat.

Before you know it, you'll be cooking entire nutritious meals in one pot. Want to make soup? Just add water or soup stock. "Soup stock" is any liquid resulting from cooking a food. You can have chicken stock, meat stock or vegetable stock. It is even possible to buy organic packaged soup stocks, just make sure to review the label.

GRAIN COOKING HINTS

Measure the grains and water into a saucepan. If you are cooking 1 cup (240 ml) of grains, use a 2-quart (2 liter) saucepan. Add 1/2 to 1 teaspoon salt if desired.

Cover the saucepan and bring to a boil over high heat. Turn the heat down to low, and steam for the recommended cooking time. Lift the lid and test the grains for tenderness. If the grains need more time, cover the saucepan and steam 5 to 10 minutes longer. If the grains need more cooking time and all the water has been absorbed, add up to 1/4 cup (60 ml) of water, cover, and continue steaming.

If tender, turn off the heat and allow the grains to rest 5 to 10 minutes before serving to fluff.

Buckwheat is the exception to the basic directions. Because the grain is so porous and absorbs water quickly, it's best to bring the water to a boil first. Then, add the buckwheat. When the water returns to a boil, cover the saucepan, turn the heat down to low, and time the steaming process.

* All grains should be washed to remove small rocks.

* Quinoa should be well rinsed in a fine strainer for 1 to 2 minutes to remove the saponins, a natural, protective coating which will give a bitter flavor if not rinsed off.

* Short grain brown rice is sometimes labeled sweet, glutinous, or sticky brown rice.

GRAINS COOKING TIMES

GRAIN (1 cup dry)	CUPS WATER	COOK TIME	CUPS YIELD
Amaranth	2 1/2	20 - 25 min.	2 1/2
Barley, pearled	3	50 - 60 min.	3 1/2
Barley, hulled	3	1 hr. 15 min.	3 1/2
Buckwheat groats *	2	15 min..	2 1/2
Millet, hulled	3 - 4	20 - 25 min.	3 1/2
Oat Groats	3	30 - 40 min.	3 1/2
Quinoa *	2	15 - 20 min.	2 3/4
Rice, brown basmati	2 1/2	35 - 40 min.	3
Rice, brown, long gr.	2 1/2	45 - 55 min.	3
Rice, brown, short grain*	2 - 2 1/2	45 - 55 min.	3
Rice, brown, quick	1 1/4	10 min.	2
Rice, wild	3	50 - 60 min.	4
Rye, berries	3 - 4	1 hr.	3
Wheat, whole berries	3	2 hrs.	2 1/2
Wheat, couscous	1	5 min.	2
Wheat, cracked	2	20 - 25 min.	2 1/4
Wheat, bulgur *	2	15 min.	2 1/2

Cooking dried beans and peas

Basic boiling

Cooking dried beans and peas is much like cooking grains except the cooking time is longer. They tend to take one-half to one hour or more, again depending on the size and density. Split peas, being small, cook much quicker than whole soy beans. Since the cooking time is long, preparing extra for re-heating is a good time and energy-saving strategy. One cup of dry beans usually requires 2 to 3 cups of water.

The basics are simple: sauce pan plus water plus beans plus lid plus heat and time.

Gourmet beans

Just as with grains, spices and other foods can be added. Pay attention to cooking times. Most other foods cook far faster than beans and don't need to be added until toward the end of the cooking cycle.

Think of your beans and peas as a medium for whatever flavor you enjoy. The difference between Southern split pea soup and Indian saffron peas is in the spices.

If you want specific ideas, ask at your favorite restaurant what they use, or consult a cook book. Your taste buds are the ultimate arbitrators of good taste.

If you're inspired to cook a grain with the bean, that's also fine, just watch your cooking times. (See the chart on page 242 for bean and pea cooking times.)

Letting up on the gas

A method for reducing the gas-forming quality of beans is to discard the first water. To do this, simply bring the beans to a boil, pour off that water and refill with cold water and start all over again bringing them to a boil, then reducing the heat to low and letting them slow boil until soft. When you discard the first water you discard many of the gas-forming elements.

Pressure cooking

Because of the high temperature involved with pressure cooking, I don't favor this type of food preparation. The higher the temperature, the more destruction of protein and loss of nutrients. Pressure cooked meals have higher carbs and lower protein than meals cooked conventionally. It's analogous to buying canned foods.

Pressure cooking does save time. Beans can be cooked in a fraction of the time. It requires a special pot with a lid that seals tight to hold in the pressure. If you decide to cook this way, consult the manual that comes with the cooker for recipes and times.

Slow cooking

Slow-cooking in a crock pot is an excellent way to prepare whole grains, dried beans and peas. These cookers use less heat over a longer time. This is more in-tune with how our ancestors cooked and it preserves more of the nutrients.

Well-organized people can start a meal in the afternoon and have it ready to eat by evening. Often when you buy a crock pot it will come with a recipe book. Consult the manufacturer's guidelines for recipes and times. Avoid models made with plastic linings; they're not only unnecessary, but unsafe.

BEANS AND PEAS COOKING TIMES

BEAN (1 cup dry)	CUPS WATER	COOK TIME	CUPS YIELD
Adzuki (Aduki)	4	45 -55 min.	3
Black Beans	4	60 -90 min	2 1/4
Black-eyed Peas	3	1 hr.	2
Cannellini (White Kidney)	3	45 min.	2 1/2
Fava Beans	3	40 -50 min.	1 2/3
Garbanzos (Chick Peas)	4	1 - 3 hrs.	2
Great Northern Beans	3 1/2	1 1/2 hrs.	2 2/3
Green Split Peas	4	45 min.	2
Yellow Split Peas	4	60-90 min.	2
Green Peas, whole	6	1 - 2 hrs.	2
Kidney Beans	3	1 hr.	2 1/4
Lentils, brown	2 1/4	45 –60 min	2 1/4
Lentils, green	2	30-45 min.	2
Lentils, red	3	20 -30 min.	2-2 1/2
Lima Beans, large	4	45 - 1 hr.	2
Lima Beans, small	4	50 -60 min.	3
Mung Beans	2 1/2	1 hr.	2
Navy Beans	3	45-60 min.	2 2/3
Pinto Beans	3	1 - 1/2 hrs.	2 2/3
Soybeans	4	3 - 4 hrs	3

BEAN AND PEA COOKING HINTS

Wash beans and discard any which are discolored or badly formed. Check for debris in the package such as small rocks or twigs and also discard them. Beans cook more quickly and their digestibility benefits with soaking in water to cover by about 3 inches (7.5 cm) for 8 hours or overnight. Discard the soak water and cook the beans in fresh water.

Soaking beans for 24 hours and changing the soak water 2 or 3 times hastens the cooking time and reduces gas.

QUICK-SOAK METHOD: When time is limited, you can wash and pick over beans and put them into a stock pot with water to cover by 3 inches (7.5 cm). Bring to a boil and boil for 10 minutes to remove toxins. Then cover and allow to soak for 1 hour. Discard soak water, add fresh water, and cook until tender.

As a general rule of thumb, 1 cup of dried beans will yield about 2 1/2 - 3 cups (.5 to .75 liters) of cooked beans.

Cooking vegetables

It's amazing how many people don't eat vegetables because they don't know how to cook them in a way that retains their flavor. Traumatized in childhood by over-cooked cafeteria vegetables, many people avoid them throughout life.

- Start with a saucepan. Add just enough water to cover the bottom.
- Add sliced, diced or chopped vegetables - the smaller the size, the quicker the cooking.
- Or, better yet, place the cut vegetables in a steamer-tray above the water.
- This is the time to add whatever spice you desire.
- Place the tight-fitting lid on top.
- Bring water to a boil. As soon as it's boiling, turn the burner to low.
- If you have cut your vegetables small or you're cooking green, leafy vegetables, you're finished as soon as the water boils. Turn off the burner and remove the pan from the heat immediately after the boiling starts.
- Dump the vegetables into a bowl or remove the steamer tray with the vegetables so they don't over-cook.
- If you are cooking harder vegetables, such as broccoli or carrots, and you haven't cut them into tiny pieces, then you may need to leave them cooking on low heat for a minute or two.
- Fork test: Vegetables are cooked when a fork can penetrate them with only a slight resistance. They are over-cooked if the fork enters without resistance.
- Shape/color test: A cooked vegetable should retain most of its basic shape and color. For instance, broccoli retains most its original green color and tree shape. On your fork it shouldn't droop or be an

anemic green.

- Don't throw out the water. It's rich in nutrients. Drink it or use it as a soup starter.
- Vegetables can be eaten plain or with a light sauce poured over them. Try a teaspoon of olive oil, a teaspoon of fresh organic lemon juice and a dash of soy sauce. There are many organic salad dressings or sauces in the market that you can sprinkle on cooked vegetables. The salad dressing described earlier can also be sprinkled on cooked vegetables. Many cultures add a light garnish of shrimp, anchovies, diced meat or other food containing protein and fat. Slivers of almonds or other nuts or seeds also add protein and fat. These combinations can become a meal in themselves.

Cooking meat, fish, and poultry

Oven-cooking is the most practical for most people. Those with super-grills and special cookers will need to consult the instruction manuals.

Baking

- Pre-heat the oven to 350° F.
- Spread a thin layer of olive oil on the inside of an oven-proof baking dish.
- Add your meat, fish or poultry in whatever size and shape you want. Again, the smaller the piece, the shorter the cooking time.
- Add whatever condiments you desire including lemon, lime, soy or tomato sauce. You may want to add diced garlic or onion.
- Place the lid on top.
- Bake until done. Time will vary on size and kind of meat. Fish generally takes 5 minutes per inch of thickness, but will vary by species. Meat, which is denser, takes longer. Test it by cutting into it and looking at the color. The more red, the more raw it is.
- Once you've done it a few times, you'll know how long the process takes. Beginners often make the mistake of over-cooking. Fish is especially delicate and needs to be watched carefully.

Poaching

Just like poaching an egg, you can cook meat in water or sauce. Simply coat your dish with olive oil and add just enough water or broth to cover the bottom of the dish. It doesn't take much. Spices, lemon and other flavor-enhancers may be added to the water. Cover with a lid to hold in the moisture. Cook as you would with baking. Coconut milk and Indonesian spices are excellent for poaching meat and fish.

Soup of the day

Soups, if done right, make nutritious meals. They only require heating water with healthy ingredients.

- Start with a saucepan.
- Add water or soup stock. Soup stock can be the liquid left over from steaming vegetables or a commercially prepared product. For instance, you can now buy organic vegetable or chicken stock. Remember to review the label.
- To the liquid, add whatever will take the longest to cook. If your soup is going to have meat or poultry, now is the time to add it. If it's going to have grains, beans or hard vegetables, they also need to go in early.
- Your cooking plan is to add the largest and hardest (densest) things first and the smaller, softer things last. This takes a little practice, but you'll catch on after a few tries. In general, beans take far longer to cook than anything else. Grains are the second-longest. Hard vegetables such as potatoes and carrots are next. Meat takes about the same time as hard vegetables. Of course this all depends on how small the vegetable and meat pieces are cut. During your early training phase use only two or three ingredients until you get the hang of it.
- Early in the cooking process, add your condiments so that their flavor will be imparted to the other ingredients. Keep it simple. Stay with what you know. Ask your mother or favorite cook what she or he uses. Garlic and onions are familiar to most people.
- Once all the harder things are cooked, add the softest things at the very end. Green leafy vegetables, since

they don't require much cooking, can be added just as you finish cooking. The residual heat will be enough.

- During the cooking process, keep the pot covered with a lid. This holds in the nutrients and, as you know, a watched pot will never boil.
- Stir the ingredients periodically to insure even cooking.
- Some people prefer to cook the ingredients in separate pans and then combine them for serving. This reduces the possibility of over or under-cooking an ingredient. I recommend this, especially for beginners.
- For an even better taste, slightly sear meats and solid vegetables such as onions, peppers, and zucchini, in a frying pan before placing them in the cooking soup. Searing is done by heating the frying pan with olive oil or butter, throwing in the food, and heating the outside of the food for 10 to 30 seconds. Just the outside is cooked. This "locks in" the flavor. The inside becomes cooked during the making of the soup.
- What kind of soup is it? Well, if you added a lot of potatoes, it's potato soup. If leeks, then its leek soup. Cabbage, carrots, beets, mutton, or chicken – it's your choice and your soup.

Meal preparation times

Excellent meals happen faster than you think. Preparing a meal generally only takes between five to 60 minutes. A fantastic salad can take five. Cooking sometimes takes longer, but steaming can be completed also in as little as five minutes.

The actual cutting, slicing and throwing in pot portion of meal preparation may take five to fifteen minutes depending on how fancy of a meal you're having and how many you're feeding.

Cooking time for grains and legumes will be 15 to 60 minutes. This is time you can spend making the salad, washing dishes, or doing something unrelated. Go change your clothes, meditate, read a poem, play with your kids, kiss your spouse (nothing more sensual than kissing to the aroma of homemade soup), stretch, call your mother, do pushups, or whatever. If you were in a restaurant or drive-through waiting for your meal, your options would be much more limited.

After the basics

Once you master boiling and baking, you're ready to buy a cookbook or accumulate recipes from family and friends. Learn to cook what you like (just don't overdo any one food - remember Variety). When you have a nice meal at a friend's house, ask for the recipe. You can sometimes ask a restaurant for their recipe, although you may want to substitute a healthier ingredient or two. Casseroles and quiches aren't as difficult as you might think.

Meal building, whether it happens in a gourmet restaurant or a tin shack is mostly about the prep work – peeling, dicing, cutting, coating dishes with oil, etcetera. If you have the right ingredients and utensils, the prep work for cooking can be done in a few minutes.

Mixing and matching

When you've done your shopping using the Three Wisdoms, you'll have a huge variety of foods to mix and match. Limitless Varieties of smells, tastes and textures await your enjoyment.

Sure it's new.
Yes, it will require new skills.
Sure it will take time.
Yes, new habits will form. Be patient and forgiving.

Let your knowledge of healthy eating and your taste buds be your guides. Soon the joy of healthy cooking will become second nature.

Chapter 21

Wisdoms in restaurants – Eating out can be healthy

Eating out can be a healthy as well as an enjoyable experience. Remember, you're in the restaurant to have a good time and enjoy a meal. Yes, you'll probably have to compromise on the quality, but that's okay, especially if you're eating well at most of your other meals.

It helps to approach restaurants like you do the grocery store - with caution. With few exceptions, most restaurants are full of health land mines. All you have to do is walk in to trip over an unhealthy food. On the other hand, there is no need to panic. Remember, in every eating situation, the first thing to do is to apply the Three Wisdoms.

Your Mantra:

"Regularly eat a Variety of Whole foods."

Common Restaurant Problems

Few cities have restaurants that use organic ingredients. Most restaurants cut corners by using inferior ingredients.

Poor quality oils are commonly used for cooking. Busy restaurants must prepare food in advance, reducing the freshness. Overcooking is common. Vegetables are often scarce. The healthiest thing you can do is eat at home, but it's fun to eat out, so go for it. Choose wisely, and remember that joy is an important food for the soul.

Regularity

How much? How often?

The first question then is when did you last eat? The answer will give you an idea of how much to eat. How much you eat will also depend on how successful your last feeding was as well as when it was. Hopefully you are already on a schedule in that you know how often your biological clock calls for you to eat. Consult Chapter 15, Regularity, if you're not clear on this basic Wisdom.

Variety: Avoiding the same old same old

Now ask yourself the second question: What have I eaten today?

The answer to this will tell you what not to eat. You want to eat a Variety of foods. If you had a chicken salad for lunch, then you don't want the same for dinner.

The second part of the variety rule is that at each meal you want carbohydrates, proteins and fats. In restaurants starchy carbohydrates and fats are in plentiful supply. The problem is the deficiency of protein and vegetables. A good approach is to start by choosing your protein, then adding the vegetable and then the rest of the carbohydrates. Fats usually take care of themselves.

Another way to increase variety if you're with another person or a group is to order several different dishes and share.

Protein First

Just like with home cooking, start by deciding on which protein to eat. If you're a vegan, your choices are somewhat limited unless it's a vegan restaurant. Vegetarians and omnivores can look for a dairy selection. Eggs can also be a good choice as long as they're not fried or scrambled because these methods cause heat and oxygen damage to the fat. Eggs should only be hard boiled, baked, poached or fried over low heat.

Chatting with the wait staff may give you some clues about the protein selection. Daily Specials are often made from fresh ingredients. Whatever they sell a lot of is also more likely to be fresh. The staff is usually willing to tell you what is freshest.

I never eat fish unless the staff swears it's fresh that day or frozen. Fish goes bad quickly. If the place doesn't specialize in seafood, they probably don't sell enough to keep it in good condition.

Lamb is often a good choice in meats because sheep are more likely to have been allowed to graze for food rather than being caged and fed grains.

Vegetables

Vegetables should be the second thing you look for in choosing your meal.

Ask the waiter how much and what kind of vegetables come with each dish you're considering. Otherwise you might end up with only sautéed onions or a sprig of parsley.

Also ask if they use fresh, canned or frozen vegetables. I know a very popular Mexican restaurant that uses the gallon cans that their vegetables and beans come in for decoration on the walls. In spite of this, many patrons still think their food is made from scratch. Simply ask.

Sometimes restaurants are happy to give you less meat and more vegetables if you request it.

Salads are often a good way to find a fresh vegetable.

However, salads with only iceberg lettuce don't provide much variety because it's mostly water and fiber. Look for exotic-sounding greens like arugala, romaine, chard and sprouts to raise your vitamin and mineral intake.

Salad caution: Always ask, especially if you have asthma and allergies, whether they treat their salad with sulfites. Some restaurants use sulfites to keep the greens looking fresher. Sulfites are a very common trigger for allergies, especially asthma.

Starches

You seldom have to worry about getting enough starch from most restaurants. There is usually way too much. Never order more than one starch. For instance, in a Mexican restaurant order rice *or* beans, not rice *and* beans unless you're a vegetarian and are counting on that combination to supply your protein. If you're already having a tamale with a thick corn wrap, you may not need any other starch.

If the restaurant serves bread, don't eat it if you're having another starch such as pasta. This is where Regularity comes in handy. If you've been eating every three to four hours, you won't be starving when they place the basket of bread or tortilla chips in front of you.

A trick to avoid eating too much starch and not enough other foods in a restaurant is to save the starch portion for last. First eat the protein and vegetables. If you're still hungry, have the starch. If you eat the starch first, you're more likely to finish it and everything else on your plate. I often leave half of my rice serving at Asian restaurants. Speaking of which, some Asian restaurants are starting to make brown rice an option. They also tend to have plenty of vegetables.

Fats

The amount of fats in most restaurant meals is usually quite sufficient, and even excessive. Unless it's an Italian restaurant that's using olive oil, most restaurants use poor-grade vegetable oils. That leaves you with two fat problems – too much and poor quality. Always ask and do the best you can.

Other restaurant suggestions

Asian restaurants will often have a choice of noodles – wheat, egg, or rice. This allows you another way to introduce Variety into your diet. And, they are very good at cooking vegetables that you may not be familiar with. Have you tried bitter melon? It's an excellent choice.

Restaurants are a good way to push yourself out of your comfort zone. Look for foods and combinations you haven't tried before. You only live once, so live it healthy.

Wholeness - Making your meal a whole lot better

You're unlikely to find organic food in a restaurant. However, you can still choose for freshness and wholeness. The wait staff will usually answer your questions, so don't be afraid to ask. You're paying for the meal so you have a right to know what's in it. One basic question regarding your forthcoming meal is, "Are the ingredients fresh, canned or frozen?" Sometimes a peek in the kitchen will tell you all you want to know.

Restaurants are compromising places. Most pizza joints will not have whole-wheat crusts or non-wheat crusts. Do the best you can with what they offer. Order lots of vegetables and a protein that is as close to natural as possible such as chicken pieces rather than sausage.

Often the salads are the only fresh food on the menu. If so, find the one with the largest variety of ingredients.

Additional Restaurant Strategies

Eat only quality appetizers

If the restaurant normally sets out a free basket of chips or bread, ask them to take it away unless they're of superior quality and taste. This avoids excessive carbohydrates and saves your appetite for more nutrient-dense foods.

If they bring out nuts or olives, depending on your appetite, you may be able to slowly eat a few.

If you're starving and must have something to eat, find out if there's something from the appetizer list that can be brought out quickly. Use this experience as a lesson. If you're too hungry to wait for your meal without chewing on the table cloth, you've waited too long or didn't eat adequately at your last feeding.

Instead of snacking on poor-quality foods use the waiting time to read, talk to your companion, freshen up in the bathroom, or contemplate your next vacation.

Too fried to handle

Fried foods are another typical downside to restaurant food. Don't let them convince you that because they use vegetable oil instead of animal fat it's good for you. It's not. In fact, it's probably worse. Vegetable oils are more susceptible to heat damage than saturated fats. (See Chapter 9, Fats 101 for more on the quality of fats.)

The sad truth is that the economic realities of the restaurant world force them to reuse frying oil for a minimum of several hours, sometimes for days. Each minute that cooking oil is exposed to heat, oxygen, and light it becomes more rancid.

Asking a few questions can make all the difference between eating well and eating excessive fat, calories and toxins.

Restaurant meals are challenging, but your Three Wisdoms mantra will prepare you for a better quality meal.

When in doubt, ask

The difference between a good meal and a bad meal can be determined by a few questions. For example:

- What are your specialties?
- Which of these comes with the most vegetables?
- Are the vegetables fresh, canned or frozen?
- Is the fish fresh or frozen?
- How big is the protein portion?

Chapter 22

Wisdoms on the go –

Powerful Snacks

First lesson: Snack is not shorthand for junk food. Too many people have the idea that the rules for snacks are different than those for meals. They eat reasonably good meals, but health takes a holiday when it comes to snacks. A bad snack can unravel a lot of the benefits of a good meal and even reduce the effectiveness of your exercise program. Snack time should not become the nutritional equivalent of a day at the carnival.

This does not mean that snacks have to be boring or unappetizing. Snacks can be nutritious, easy to carry and tasty, without being too salty, sweet, fatty or adulterated with chemicals. Most people find their taste perception matures as they change their eating habits. What they once thought was desirable often become too sweet and "chemical tasting." Healthy snacks grow to be desirable, partly because you learn to enjoy the taste and partly because you feel better when eating better.

The fact is that for most people taste has little to do with the flavors being picked up by the receptors on the tongue. Taste buds are only one part of a constellation of perceptions. Temperature, texture, creaminess, crunchiness, smell, stickiness, color, and what the food industry calls "mouth feel" are all sensations that make up the eating experience. You didn't think that the food industry was adding all those artificial colors, thickening agents, odors and texture enhancers for their own aesthetic pleasure, did you? It's all part of research, development and marketing.

Your sensations of eating have been trained to jump through hoops designed by the food and beverage industry. Forget any naive ideas you might have about

> *"Sugar and salt are the enemies of taste (as well as health)."*

manufactured foods being "natural." Even the modern apple has been engineered to taste and feel differently from its ancestors. If you want a natural taste experience, chew on pine needles.

This is not to say that your snacks will consist of pine needles and crab apples, but I think it is important for you to realize you have been programmed to eat certain foods, and that you can take control of your food sensations. For many people a healthy snack may mean really tasting something for the first time rather than just gulping down a sugary drink.

Sugar and salt are the enemies of taste (as well as health). After tasting little else since birth, many people have adapted to only tasting sugar and salt. Any subtle distinction in tastes is lost under the load of these two cheap commodities. For example, think of the difference between the cold, tangy, effervescence of a cola, and a room-temperature, day-old cola. Some find the former a taste sensation and use the latter for putting out their cigarette butts. It's the same product either way. Sugar gives you the rush, but it is carried on a magic carpet of bubbly illusion.

When trying new foods, keep your mind and taste buds open. Sure, you may have to experiment, but the chances are good you'll find many new foods you'll enjoy.

The wonderful thing about **Nutrition-1-2-3** is that the same nutritional rules apply to meals and snacks -

Regularity, Variety and Wholeness. Don't eat snacks that steal the steel you've built with your healthy meals.

Remember the proteins, carbs and fats

You'll find you feel better if your snacks, just like your meals, contain protein, carbs and fats. I know it's tempting to just have an apple or muffin - and they are stomach-filling - but they don't fill your nutritional reserves or keep your hormones in balance. That takes eating a balance of nutrients.

The Cheese does not stand alone- Variety!

Most single foods do not give you the balance of protein, starch and fat you need. A solo piece of cheese has protein and fat, but little starch. An apple has the starch, but little protein and fat. This means you need to mix cheese with an apple; or, celery and chicken; or, an egg and salad. Nuts, seeds and beans are the closest to being a healthy mixture of protein, starch and fat.

Fruit and vegetables, not
crackers and cookies

Notice how in my examples above I don't mention bread and crackers? Most of us get plenty of these kinds of starches already. Snacks offer you an opportunity to get more of the nutritional value of fruits and vegetables without many calories. The exception to this would be the person doing hard manual labor who needs more calories.

Protein bars and other temptations

In this busy world where we often find ourselves away from the safety of our own kitchen, it's helpful (and some would say lifesaving) to have an easy-to-carry, nutritious snack bar.

As a service to my patients I have spent time surveying "protein" and "health" bars. There must be a need, because there's a glut of them on the market. However well they fit a market niche, for the most part I've been disappointed in what I've seen.

When shopping for snacks, read labels carefully. Here are some guidelines.

Not enough protein in the "protein" bar

Rarely do I find a bar that has a favorable ratio of starch, protein and fat. You want to look for a protein bar that has a macro-nutrient composition close to hunter-gatherer standards and consistent with modern research on glucose control. That translates into something in the neighborhood of 40 percent carbs, 30 percent protein and 30 percent fat calories.

The easiest way to orient yourself to a label is to start with the protein content. Let's say the bar has 15 grams of protein. Next look at the carbohydrates. If your goal is a ratio of 40 percent carbohydrate to 30 percent protein, then you want about 20 grams of carbohydrates to balance with the 15 grams of protein. If the bar contains 30 grams of protein, then there should be 40 grams of carbs. These ratios do not have to be exact so ballpark estimates are fine.

Most bars I've seen are in an entirely different neighborhood - the street of high carbs. I commonly see bars that contain 30 grams of carbs and 10 grams of protein or a 30/10 ratio. That's a prescription for high insulin, blood sugar and weight gain and all the problems that go along with these.

Don't leave out the (good!) fat

The fat component of a snack is just as important as the protein and starch. Quality is the most important factor, but percentage is also important.

Remember, your general goal is 40 percent carbs, 30 percent protein and 30 percent fat.

A typical bar is the one with 30 grams of carbs, 10 grams of protein and 20 grams of fat. The percentage of calories would then be 30/10/40 (carbs/protein/fat). These very unhealthy ratios are typical of snack bars.

The ideal bar to achieve our theoretically perfect ratio will contain something like 20 grams of carbs, 15 grams of protein and 7 grams of fat (40/30/30). Or some multiple of these like 40 grams of carbs, 30 grams of protein and 15 grams (30 calories) of fat. This equals the ideal 40/30/30 ratio of macro-nutrients.

You'll find it difficult to find a bar that has exactly this ratio, but you can get close. These numbers don't need to be exact. Also, as an individual who is exercising regularly you may find that your ratio of carbohydrates needs to be a little higher. Maybe you function better on more protein. Figuring out your personal ratios is where Regularity comes in.

Mixing bars with food

Since most bars tend to be too high in carbs, you can make up for this by adding something with protein. For instance, there are some very good all-natural fruit bars available. Fruit is a source of carbs, vitamins and minerals, but has little protein or fat. So, you could eat a hard-boiled organic egg containing protein and fats with a fruit bar. Or a handful of almonds (protein and fat) with a fruit bar. A slice of smoked salmon or a piece of cheese would also balance nicely with a fruit bar, just as it would balance a piece of fruit.

Yuck to hydrogenated oils, additives and preservatives

Unfortunately, most "health" bars contain cheap, health-robbing hydrogenated oils. If you see something like "partially hydrolyzed vegetable oil" listed on the label, return the bar to the shelf and call in a hazardous-waste crew to haul it away.

The ill effects of hydrogenated oils are so well known that even the FDA, major nutrition groups and the new food pyramid have started warning consumers against eating them. I suppose it's better late than never.

The same is true of additives and preservatives. You don't need them and you will do better without them.

It is extremely difficult to find a bar without bad oils, preservatives and additives, so read the labels carefully.

Type of protein

Another issue with bars is the source of protein. One concern here is if you have allergies. Soy and peanuts are used often because they're cheap. They also are of the lowest quality and highest allergic potential. Rice protein is the least likely allergy inducer. Whey is the most biologically available, highest quality protein. Whey is the liquid protein that separates out from the curd when milk sits. The milk solids (powdered milk) used in bars are often of low quality. And remember that dairy is a common allergen.

My favorite bars

BioGenesis Neutraceuticals, Inc., out of Mill Creek, Washington (near Seattle), makes the only bars I know of that have the 40/30/30 ratio, have no hydrogenated oil, use organic ingredients and even give you a nice supply of vitamins.

They make several flavors, including ones made with

organic chocolate and natural vanilla. (Most companies use chemically manufactured vanillin.) For those on higher-protein diets, they also make a line of bars with a higher protein content and lower carbs.

I like that they are not super-sweet when compared with commercial bars. This helps people lose their sweet tooth.

Lara Bars and several other companies make bars that are simply fruit and nuts mixed. That means you're eating a healthy combination of protein, fat and carbs with each bar.

Snack size

How large your snack is depends on your needs. Most of us with sedentary jobs don't need much. If you're too hungry – jittery and nervous – at your meal, you could use a snack a few hours earlier.

Examples of health snacks

- A half a piece of fruit and a wedge of cheese.
- A few celery sticks and a piece of chicken.
- One handful of nuts contains protein, starch and fat. Avoid roasted and salted nuts.
- A protein shake or bar. A shake does not have to have milk at all but may use yogurt, dilute fruit juice or even water as its liquid base. There are some excellent whey or rice protein shakes available that taste good hand-shaken with water so no blender is required.
- Almond butter on a wedge of apple or stick of celery.
- A fruit bar with a protein source such as nuts, cheese, chicken, or smoked fish.

Note all of these suggestions contain protein, carbohydrate and fat – a variety of macronutrients. The rule of thumb for how often and how large a snack should be is to consume just enough to get you through to the next meal without feeling stuffed or overly hungry.

You'll know if your snack was adequate at your next meal. If you're starving, nervous and irritable, then your snack wasn't adequate in size or proportions.

Oh, please don't think me a nag, but remember Variety. Don't fall into the habit of having the same snack every day.

Enjoy!

SECTION V

Wisdoms to the Rescue-

Preventing and Treating Common Health Problems

Chapter 23

Medicine for the 21st Century –

Treat with the plate, not the prescription pad

It might sound strange in light of some of my earlier comments, but I feel fortunate to be part of this modern world of high-tech gadgets, biotechnology, and the unraveling of our genetic code.

Some people think that naturopathic medicine is stuck in the past, relying on old herbal texts, spirituality, and ancient wisdoms. What's exciting about naturopathy is that it was born in the past, but continues to be nurtured in the present. I like to say that naturopathy is the best of traditional medicine supported by modern scientific research.

Let's look at a patient with joint pain, for instance. (We won't load her condition with fear by labeling it with a Latin word such as arthritis, which simply means joint inflammation.) In the past a good natural doctor in the Americas, Europe, India, Africa or Asia would have prescribed massage, moderate exercise, and natural anti-inflammatories such as foods rich in omega-3 oils and herbs such as boswelia and turmeric.

The patient likely would have recovered and without

side effects. This is what I'd call the best of ancient traditions. They worked in the past and they still work today. Also, many traditional therapies are supported by scientific research on the effects of foods and herbs in modifying inflammation.

Certainly there would have been other treatments available in the past, some of them not helpful and perhaps even harmful. After all, this was a time of empirical science - trial and error. Nothing was known about how these therapies worked on a biochemical level. Often spirits or gods were believed to be the arbitrator of wellness and disease. Through millennia of this trial and error medicine, many very effective therapies were developed and written down.

> *"What's exciting about naturopathy is that it was born in the past, but continues to be nurtured in the present. I like to say that naturopathy is the best of traditional medicine supported by modern scientific research."*

It's easy to lose sight of our past medical successes and realize how new our current medical system is. Think about something as basic as a microscope. The microscope had to be invented before we could discover bacteria which led to an entire field of study called microbiology. In just the last few hundred years the circulation of the blood was discovered. Vitamins have been known for less than 100 years. New properties of blood, new vitamins, and new bacteria are continually being discovered.

Part of the benefit of our new discoveries (from the microscope to the MRI imager) and our new fields of research (from microbiology to biotechnology) is the answer to "Why?"

In just the relatively short time I've been in practice, since 1982, thousands of answers to questions about why the body responds to certain foods or herbs in particular ways have been discovered. One food may increase the functioning of the thyroid gland while another helps the liver detoxify poisons. Ancient doctors knew about these herbs, but not why they worked. For example, now that we know the chemicals involved in inflammation, we can measure their response to foods and herbs in alleviating joint pain.

Yes, most of the research money goes into discovering drugs, but the side-benefit of modern science has been the answer to many of the "Why?" questions in natural medicine.

Why Medicine

You might ask your own "Why?" question: Why does it matter if the cure is a drug or a food?

One very big reason: Most drugs are aimed at blocking symptoms, not curing the underlying condition. In our example of the patient with joint pain, her choice is between a drug that blocks the inflammation but also blocks her body's natural healing responses and often causes side effects, or a food that nourishes her own healing response. After all, the body has evolved its own anti-inflammatory system over millions of years, so why not use it? My vote is for the cure that works with the body's evolution, not for a drug cooked up in a lab.

I call natural medicine "Why medicine". We ask "Why?" as we seek answers to treat the cause.

Bringing medical thinking up to date

A common complaint against our dominant medical system is that it's impersonal. The excuse is that we pay the price of lost personal interactions for the benefits of technology. But I feel the loss of the personal is not because of technology but because of the way it's applied.

Medicine continues to function predominantly under the 19th Century model of Henry Ford's production line. If a doctor thinks that every person is the same and sees her job as removing and replacing parts, then she's apt to quickly lose any personal relationship to the patient. I witnessed this process many times when I worked in hospitals; the young idealistic medical-school graduate pounded by long hours and the relentless emphasis on drugs became a prescription-writing robot.

Questions like, "Why is this person in pain?" become buried under tight schedules and pharmaceutical indoctrination. It's no wonder that physicians have such high rates of alcohol and drug abuse. They're caring people who have lost sight of their patients as individuals and the ability to ask "Why?"

Actually, Henry Ford and cars are not an entirely appropriate analogy, since most people pay more attention to their cars than their health and mechanics usually cannot cover up symptoms but must find the cause of a problem before administering the cure.

> "This is the future of medicine:
> * Technology at the service of wholistic medicine.
> * Therapies that work with, rather than against the body.
> *Seeing each person as unique.
> * Treating the person as an integrated whole.
> * Knowing that true cure means truly caring."

Fortunately, much of science, if not medicine, has moved beyond the Model T and the 19th Century model. Good scientists are not only accelerating our understanding of the nuts and bolts of human physiology, but envisioning how all the parts fit together and interact. This is essential support for wholistic medicine.

This is the future of medicine: Technology at the service of wholistic medicine. Therapies that work with, rather than against the body. Seeing each person as unique. Treating the person as an integrated whole. Knowing that true cure means truly caring.

I feel privileged to be part of a profession in which I can witness "miracles" every day. Talk to any doctor that relies on nutrition and natural therapies and you'll hear stories of 'incurable" diseases responding to the simplest of dietary changes. Why? Because we take the time to ask "Why?"

If you're broken, find a cure

In diet, as with many things in life, the old adage applies, "If it ain't broke, don't fix it."

If you consistently feel great, don't catch colds, haven't been diagnosed with a disease, are symptom free, and do not use any over-the-counter or prescription medications, you may not need to change how you eat. However, this state of optimal health is rare in our polluted, high-stress, and nutrient-depleted world.

Most Americans do have health problems. Even those patients that come to my office for a routine physical exam and claim to be problem free usually will admit to having something not quite right. It's a rare person who can fill out a thorough health history without marking a few symptoms. Sometimes they've lived with a condition for so long they ignore it. This is quite common with skin problems such as eczema and minor aches and pains. Sometimes it's a problem that the patient has been led to believe there is no cure for. Premenstrual misery is a common problem for many women who don't realize it's completely treatable. Same goes for arthritis – many people think it's genetic and suffer needlessly.

Acid reflux, constipation, gas and bloating are also symptoms that people live with without knowing that these are actually signs of a system out of balance. Or, a person may have been taking an over-the-counter medication to control their indigestion, rash or pain for so long that it has become a routine part of their life. They've never stopped to realize they have a health problem that would be better addressed at its cause, not just hidden behind a medication that may be eroding their health in other ways.

Older people often chalk their symptoms up to aging. In my experience, people have been feeling older at younger and younger ages. How does a 30 or even 40 year old blame their knee pain on "getting old" when people twice their age are running marathons? Most of the symptoms associated with aging have been shown to have more to do with lack of exercise and poor diet than the ticking of a clock.

This brings up the "genetic" excuse: "My parents had (fill in the blank) so it makes sense I'm having (fill in the symptom)." It's very sad to see people who have resigned themselves to pain and misery of various kinds because they think it's a genetic problem. Lifestyle, especially exercise and diet, trumps genetics 90 percent of the time.

Yes, most of us have some symptoms and mostly they can be reduced or eliminated if treated correctly. The patients that claim to be completely symptom-free are usually either in deep denial or very young.

Food is forever

Many things affect your health. Food, however, is forever. Although other lifestyle choices influence your health, it's usually not as seriously as diet.

Some dangers, such as air pollution and smoking, are unavoidable. But food is controllable. It is something you have a great amount of power over. How you eat is a health decision you make every day.

Some might argue that smoking, excessive alcohol or taking illicit drugs have more of an impact on people's lives than diet. And for a minority of people, that's true. What a heavy smoker, drinker or drug addict eats probably doesn't have as much impact on their health as does their negative habit. On the other hand, if they eat an excellent diet along with their bad habit, the quality and quantity of their life will not degenerate as rapidly. Excellent scientific research shows that a good diet can reduce the consequences of unhealthy life choices. If the person only has a light bad habit, diet may make all the difference in the world. Of course the outcome of addictive behavior depends on other factors including genetics, duration of habit, combination of habits, and other factors.

For the majority of us who don't smoke, drink alcohol to excess, or take drugs, our day-in and day-out eating and exercise habits are the most significant health factors in our lives.

You could also argue that a person's safety decisions - such as the use of car seatbelts and bicycle helmets - are the most important health decisions. I agree that safety devices should be used. For a relatively small minority of people these precautions significantly influence their health and welfare. Safety measures may mean the difference between life and death. And they may mean the difference between health and disability. Not using them increases your chances of not being healthy or alive. On the other hand, most people (fortunately) go through their lives never having their life depend on a seatbelt. They reduce their risk of injury IF they are in an accident by wearing one, but they've never been in an accident. Seatbelts may save your life, but good nutrition will definitely improve its quality.

Nutrition is different. It's not an either/or, accident or/no accident, situation. Eating a poor quality diet will influence your health every day, every minute, even when you're sleeping. Every bite of food you take either adds to or subtracts from your health.

This section discusses specific health problems and the positive way they're influenced by diet. Diabetes, heart disease, cancer, stroke, mental illness, thyroid, digestive problems, asthma, hormone imbalances, and arthritis are only a few of the conditions that are known, by scientific research, to be impacted by diet.

Chapter 24

Energy Wisdoms –

Are you suffering an energy crisis?

Pam: unrecognized energy problem

"Is this true?" I asked Pam, a glum woman in her thirties. "Do you really drink six cups of coffee a day?" I was pointing to the diet form she'd filled out before her first visit.

"Yes, I have a busy life." She said this matter-of-factly, like this explained her large coffee intake. We'd already talked about her main reasons for coming in - headaches and alternating constipation and diarrhea.

"Let's go back to this question about your energy. You wrote your average energy level is nine out of ten. How would you rate it if you didn't drink coffee?"

"I don't know. Maybe a two or three? I never go without it."

The energy crisis at home

Statistically, fatigue is cited as the most common reason for seeking medical advice. I certainly see a lot of people with this complaint. I'm also amazed how many people don't think about their energy until I've asked.

I've had hundreds of patients who will say their energy is good or average, but upon questioning, they admit they don't have the energy to do more than is minimally necessary. In other words, they just "get by."

They get up and go to work and in the evening have enough energy to watch TV. There are other things they want to do, but they never get around to them. Often these people don't even know it's possible to feel more energetic. Some, like Pam, self-medicate with coffee.

If getting by is all you aspire to, then maybe your diet is good enough. However, if you want to feel more vital and energetic, to have more stamina and end-of-the-day reserves, the Three Wisdoms may help you.

Energy Evaluation

The first stop in your search for more energy should be a doctor's office. You want to make sure you don't have any obvious health problems such as anemia, diabetes, or low thyroid - to name just the most common.

I suggest you see a professional who is health oriented. There are plenty of disease-oriented doctors who will do a simple screening of your blood and a quick once-over physical exam. This can be helpful if you have any obvious disease, but inadequate for a person who has "vertical disease."

Is your disease vertical or horizontal?

A person has "vertical disease" if he or she is outwardly healthy and has no obvious health problems, but doesn't feel good. Her physical exam and laboratory tests are normal, but she knows she used to have more get up and go. Often, on closer examination, she will have subtle physical changes that go unnoticed or are considered "normal" to a physician who is not practicing wholistic medicine. Most MDs focus on "horizontal disease" – illnesses that keep you bedridden or even in the hospital.

In "vertical disease", she feels like, as one patient told me, "I can't complain about anything specific. It's like I can't press the gas pedal all the way to the floor."

Most MDs are good enough to find "horizontal disease" and their solution is to write a prescription - but they are inadequately trained to find "vertical disease." Most likely, if you complain of fatigue and your doctor can't find any blood abnormalities, he or she will suggest you see a psychiatrist or, more common these days, write you a prescription for an anti-depressant.

It might be true; you may need to see someone about depression (for counseling, not for drugs!), but doctors who practice this way are missing out on the opportunity to help the majority of their patients.

Dawn of the half-dead

While it's very rewarding to help a patient recover from a life-threatening illness, I have found that some of my most rewarding cases are those patients who have been rescued from a life of half-living, of being chronically tired and unable to fulfill their ambitions - the woman who wants to start her own business, the man who can't move out of his rut at work, the young mother who wants to be a better parent. The majority of people fall into the category of "vertical disease" and there is help for most of them.

First of all, your doctor needs to follow a basic lesson from medical school: treat the patient, not the lab report. Laboratory testing is important, but is only a guideline. The report may have all the correct numbers, but it's the patient who isn't feeling well. If they say they don't feel well, believe them and not the test results.

To help solve the problem of the patient who is outwardly healthy, but inwardly sick, I find it helpful to employ a number of additional tools besides blood, urine and physical exam. I employ a comprehensive health screening questionnaire. This requires the patient answer several hundred questions related to his or her health. These can then be evaluated, either by hand or computer, for the doctor's use in categorizing symptoms. For example, the patient's answers may lead me to focus on improving the patient's digestive function, or her immune system, or ability to detoxify environmental toxins. Sometimes it gives clues that reveal the need for more detailed laboratory testing. The comprehensive health questionnaire is a useful tool in evaluating a patient's overall health.

These questions help us decide if there is an energy problem and, if so, if it's related to food, blood sugar, sleep,

Fourteen Energy Questions

In addition to the Comprehensive Health Questionnaire, I ask all my patients a few basic energy questions:

1. Rate your average daily energy on a zero to ten scale. Zero is dead. Ten is a Jack La Lanne (my hero).
2. When is your energy the lowest during the day?
3. When is your energy the highest?
4. How does your energy change (up or down) with eating?
5. Do you have any problems falling asleep at night?
6. How many hours do you sleep?
7. What time do you go to bed and what time do you wake?
8. Do you sleep through the night?
9. Do you wake feeling rested?
10. Do you nap or would you like to nap during the day?
11. Do you exercise? What kind and how often?
12. How does exercise affect your energy?
13. Do you rely on stimulants such as coffee or caffeinated soft drinks to get you through the day?
14. Do you have the energy to do what you want to do with your life?

exercise or other lifestyle factors. It also gives us a baseline for measuring the success of treatment.

Most people don't remember what they told me at the first appointment. So if they say, "I'm not getting any better. My energy scale is at six." I can remind them that, although they have a ways to go, at their first visit they rated their energy level as three out of ten.

These questions can also alert patients to lifestyle factors. If they see, for instance, that they do feel better on the days they exercise, they are more inclined to continue exercising. Likewise, sleep is often an undervalued health activity.

Diet/symptom diary

Another helpful tool is a detailed diet/symptom survey. The patient writes down everything eaten and all symptoms for a week or two then reviews it with the doctor. This can sometimes reveal the source of an energy problem.

It's not uncommon, for instance, for a person to discover that his or her energy is affected by certain foods or combinations of foods or by not eating for long periods of time. I have seen the diet/symptom diary answer significant health mysteries. The "Ah ha!" factor may not be rocket science, but it does reflect on a person's biochemical make-up.

Energy and weight gain

A person's energy level and their weight are often linked. Many patients, upon reflection, recognize that their body weight started creeping up when the energy level started going down.

If you're putting on weight and can't seem to exercise enough, maybe it's because you don't have enough energy.

Swinging Low

Some patients find that their energy has wide swings throughout the day. They may jump out of bed raring to go, but spend their afternoons in a delirious funk. Or, they may not fully wake up until noon, and then feel great for a couple of hours before they burn out. Others find themselves on a continuous roller coaster of highs and lows without any detectable pattern.

> *"Two of the most common reasons for the energy rollercoaster are blood sugar fluctuations and hormone swings."*

Two of the most common reasons for the energy rollercoaster are blood sugar fluctuations and hormone swings. Blood sugar, insulin, glucagon (a hormone that "balances" insulin), cortisol and adrenalin (both stress hormones) have powerful effects on mood and energy. The Three Wisdoms, especially Regularity and Wholeness, can correct these ups and downs.

Diet and Energy

While there are many things that affect energy, the most common cause of low energy is a dietary weakness. I've seen thousands of otherwise healthy people transform their energy levels with simple dietary changes.

Very often patients with "vertical disease" can learn a great deal about themselves as well as cure their energy problem by going on a test diet.

By simply (theoretically simple but often difficult in practice) changing your diet for one month you may experience profound changes. Some patients choose to do a radical change, especially if they're eating an unhealthy diet. Others prefer a gradual approach and change things a little at a time.

Jeff: Unrecognized fatigue

A recent patient, Jeff, who had originally consulted with me about his acne, came back after one week of changing his diet, which simply involved eating a good breakfast, and said, "I didn't realize my energy was so low. I feel one thousand percent better."

Of course, not everyone will feel "one thousand percent better" but wouldn't it be great to feel 50 percent better? Or even ten percent? If you live to be 70 years old, ten percent more energy is like adding seven years to your life. The added energy might be just enough to get you up off the couch and out to a community or PTA meeting. What about that hobby you've been neglecting while you've been sitting watching TV or surfing the net?

I would encourage anyone with an energy problem to follow the Three Wisdoms diet for one month. You will decrease your chances of cardiovascular disease, cancer, diabetes and all of the most common complaints of our time and, chances are, you will also improve your energy level.

Energy to burn

If you don't have the vitality you think you should, do something about it. After ruling out horizontal medical conditions, look at your diet.

You don't have to read a dozen books or follow a fad diet. The answer to your energy problem may be as simple as doing what your distant ancestors did: follow the Three Wisdoms.

Chapter 25

Anti-aging Wisdoms –

Too old too early?

James: old before his time

"I suppose it's inevitable," James joked as he pinched his spare tire. "My blood pressure and cholesterol are high normal. My doctor wants me to start on meds. I came to you to see if there was an herb or something I could take instead, at least for a few years." He laughed as he added, "What bugs me the most are my knees are giving out. I know I'm getting old, almost forty, but I'd like to slow it down a bit."

Lessons from the old

I'm continually shocked by how many relatively young people believe they're "getting old." Some of them haven't hit the big three-O! Others in their fifties and sixties talk like they're lucky to be alive at their "advanced age." Too many people see putting on weight, creaky knees, and other symptoms as inevitable signs of aging.

When I started in naturopathic practice in 1982 I was lucky enough to inherit a few patients from an older naturopath, Dr. Carroll, who had recently died. What amazed me was how many of them were in their 70s and 80s and still living quite vibrant lives. A few hadn't been to an MD in many years. Some were the adult children of Dr. Carroll's early patients – who also had never been to an MD. Most of them never took prescription drugs or even over-the-counter medicines. As a young doctor, these patients inspired my belief in naturopathic medicine and the power of the body's innate healing abilities.

I know we all age. However, I also know that we have a great influence on how we age and what sort of diseases we'll suffer from as we age.

Isn't it normal to feel old in middle age?

No. Not in the natural world.

Yes, the young do have more flexibility when it comes to diet. Their youth can get them through a lot of bad meals. Eventually, however, side effects begin to show. By their 30s they're complaining of "middle-age" symptoms such as arthritis, high blood sugar, excessive weight and even heart disease. Sad to say, many people accept their premature decline as if there was nothing to do about it. Middle-age decline is not inevitable or irreversible.

When scientists look at humans who live in traditional cultures and eat a diet similar to what their ancestors ate in Paleolithic times, they do not see a middle-age decline. These people tend to live healthy, productive lives until old age, and then decline rapidly into death.

The same is true in animal studies. Animals eating their native diets tend to live in good health until old age, not declining until just before death. Zoo and domestic animals that are eating non-traditional diets go through the same middle-age decline as most humans. They develop arthritis, diabetes, cancer and heart disease.

Why the premature decline?

There are, of course, many factors involved. I wouldn't want to underestimate such things as stress, lack of exercise and the millions of tons of pollution modern humans are subjected to. However, since this book is about nutrition, I'll focus on that.

The farther our diets shift from the Three Wisdoms, the worse our health becomes. Encouragingly, when people substitute "meals of steel" for "meals that steal", their health always improves.

A very large research project, the Hanes II Nutrition Study, showed that 50 percent of the U.S. population was below the recommended dietary allowance (RDA) for some vitamins and minerals. This total diet study, conducted from 1982-1988 and published in the *Journal of the American Dietetic Association*, found that intakes of calcium, magnesium, iron, zinc and copper were on average below the estimated safe and adequate daily dietary intake.

A 1997 California Department of Health survey showed that two-thirds of the respondents did not consume enough fruits and vegetables.

There are many similar studies to cite and all are indications that the average diet gets worse every year.

Even those of you who eat what I call the "not bad" diet - avoiding fast foods - need to consider what the *Journal of Applied Nutrition* reported in 1993. The researchers found that organic produce had 90 percent more nutrients than commercially-raised foods. If you realize that what people ate for millions of years was all organic and that it has only been in the last 100 years that non-organic foods became available, then you might decide that a "not bad" diet isn't so great after all.

Can a poor diet make you feel old?

It most certainly can. Numerous studies have associated the modern industrial diet with premature aging and a host of chronic diseases. Some of the most dramatic of these studies are the ones that follow a population after they immigrate into U.S. culture. For instance, Japanese people who move to the U.S. and consume the Standard American Diet (SAD) foods quickly see their cholesterol and blood pressures rising.

In my clinic I have seen many patients reverse the downward trend toward premature aging by applying the Three Wisdoms.

Chapter 26

Weight Wisdoms –

Weight-Loss for Life

Volumes have been written in the scientific and lay literature about the problem of excess weight and obesity in the U.S. Everyone agrees excess weight is an epidemic that kills. It is associated with all of the major killing diseases of our times including heart disease, cancer, stroke and diabetes.

Sandra –
Gaining weight while eating "right"

"I do everything right." Sandra started her consultation sounding defiant. "I exercise heavily four to six hours a week. My diet is impeccable 95 percent of the time. But I can't lose any weight and if I stray by one calorie," she now sounded wounded, "I gain weight. It's not fair."

She then went on to describe the numerous weight-loss programs she'd undertaken over the last twenty years. Each one had been temporarily successful, yet impossible to maintain. The result being that she was forty pounds overweight. "Why am I such a failure?"

"It is unfair," I said. "And you're not a failure. What you've been doing to lose weight is the failure. What you were told to do was wrong. My observation is that you're an intelligent person who's motivated and takes concrete actions for her health. That's highly commendable. Unfortunately, you fell into the same trap as millions. The low calorie, low fat diet has a ninety-five percent failure rate. When you change to a winning strategy, you'll lose weight."

What is obesity and overweight?

Overweight is generally defined as a Body Mass Index (BMI) above 25. A BMI above 30 is obese, although some authors use 28. Your BMI is a calculation based on your height and weight. (See Section IX for chart on BMI.)

For example, a person who is 5'3" and weighs 140 pounds has a BMI of 25. At 170 pounds, a person of the same height has a BMI of 30. A person who is 5'8" has a BMI of 25 if they weigh 165 pounds or a BMI of 30 if they weigh 195 pounds.

Other common methods of estimating a person's body fat are skin-fold thickness and bio-impedance (electrical resistance) measurements. Skin-fold thickness is difficult to measure and best left to experts. Bio-impedance measures the percentage of body fat by sending an electrical impulse through your body. It's smart enough to separate fat from muscle. Hand-held bio-impedance devices are now available in drug stores for less than $50. You can also find them built into scales.

BMI and bio-impedance in combination with weight are excellent ways to track your health. Weight alone can fool you, since some people are of normal weight, but have a high percentage of fat. A very muscular person, in contrast, might look very unhealthy to a scale. Bio-impedance can tell you to within a few percentage points just how much of you is fat and how much is muscle.

Why the baby boom?
Common denominators of weight gain:

- Greater consumption of processed, high-calorie foods = Failing the Wholeness Wisdom.
- Decreased consumption of fruits and vegetables = Failing the Variety Wisdom.
- Missing meals, especially breakfast = Omitting the Regularity Wisdom.
- A sedentary lifestyle = Forgetting the "move or die" axiom.

Fat does not bequeath fat

Contrary to common misconceptions, total fat consumption may not be a major factor in creating an obese world. In the past 20 years the U.S. population has reduced fat intake by 14 percent, yet we are 32 percent fatter. The consumption of sugar and refined carbohydrates, which was up by 110 percent in the same period, are a much greater problem than excessive fat for the majority of people in this country.

The average American is getting one-quarter to one-third of their calories from sugar. Soda consumption averages 40 gallons per person per year. Teenagers average 3.33 cans of soda each day. These villains far outstrip naturally-occurring fat in food as a cause of obesity.

The weight of the evidence (if you'll pardon my pun) is in. People are increasingly overweight and obese because they are consuming more calorie-rich, nutrient-poor foods. It is the increased popularity of modern processed foods, plus the lack of exercise, that is fattening our adults and children which increases their disease rates and while shortening their lives. It is a national and international health problem of the first order.

If you are overweight or obese, you will benefit greatly from applying the Three Wisdoms.

Diets don't work

The ineffectiveness of short-term dieting has been proven time and again. Unfortunately, most people don't know this and thousands, like Sandra, keep trying and failing to lose weight by cutting back on calories for a few days or a few weeks.

> *"This cycle of "yoyo" dieting – down a few, up a few more, down, up, up and up – has resulted in overweight people becoming obese."*

Millions of dollars are spent on "new" diets and "special" foods. Millions of pounds are lost, and then quickly regained – plus a few more pounds to remind you that you failed. This cycle of "yoyo" dieting – down a few, up a few more, down, up, up and up – has resulted in overweight people becoming obese.

The only proven way to lose weight and keep it off is through actively changing the way you exercise and eat every day of your life. Sorry, no miracle cures. The body doesn't work that way. It needs balanced nutrition and regular exercise. This does not necessarily mean a radical change in eating habits. It might mean something as simple as adding one meal (breakfast) or one healthy food (vegetables) to your eating schedule. Whatever makes the difference for you must be done consistently and not just as a temporary fix.

With calories, quality trumps quantity

Yes, excessive calories, whether they are from protein, starch or fat, will lead to increased weight gain. Controlling the number of calories you consume is important. However, the question for most people is: how do I cut calories and not go crazy and break into a bakery and eat everything in sight?

A thorough understanding of the research and physiology of weight loss leads to the conclusion that, for most people, the quality of the calories consumed makes a critical difference in how many calories they will eat in a day. Poor quality intake leads to higher overall intake. Good quality reduces quantity.

Proteins and fats of the highest quality are less likely to contribute to obesity. Whole, natural foods that are full of vitamins, nutrients and omega-3 fats are going to help you lose weight. This is not because they have fewer calories, but because the high quality and nutrient density reduces your hunger for empty calories.

I rarely suggest that my patients restrict calories. Most overweight people have already tried and failed to lose weight by watching caloric intake. I find it more useful to have them not worry about what they're leaving out, but to get excited about what they're adding to their diet.

A person following the Three Wisdom plan doesn't need to worry about restricting their intake of calories because they've added a Variety of Whole foods at Regular intervals. As the quality of their diet improves, the quantity diminishes. Oh, and with the new shape of their body they also feel more energetic.

Wholistic approach to weight loss

Naturopathic physicians approach weight quite differently than the dominant medical-industrial-complex. We look at excess weight not as a fat problem, but as a health problem.

Many things influence why one person will be a healthy weight while another is literally dying from obesity. While the specifics of our approach are individualized to each patient, there are a few general rules that apply to most people.

The basics of weight loss

There are a number of strategies for weight loss and improved body composition that everyone can apply. If these strategies are not working for you, then I suggest you seek the help of a physician trained in healthy weight management.

1. Regularity

- Determine a regular feeding schedule that works best for you and stick with it.
- Avoid going more than 3 to 4 hours without at least a small healthy snack.
- If at mealtime you find yourself craving sweets, feeling ravenously hungry, jittery or otherwise falling apart, evaluate your last meal or snack for mistakes.
- Eat a breakfast containing protein.

2. Wholeness and Variety

- Concentrate on improving the quality and variety of your diet, not reducing the quantity.
- Eating more whole foods will reduce your desire for empty calories.
- Limit calories only by limiting junk food.
- Don't limit your food choices, expand them with more Variety. Your choices must be healthy ones. Remember Wholeness.
- Every feeding should include a Variety of protein, carbohydrates, and fat.

3. Drink 8 glasses of water a day

Most weight-loss diets recommend water as an important tool. Research in the *Journal of Clinical Endocrinology and*

Metabolism, (December 2003) showed that water intake increases the rate at which people burn calories. A little over two cups of water a day increased metabolism by an amazing 30 percent. It is estimated that by consuming 1.5 liters of water a day the average person would burn an extra 17,400 calories a year, for a weight loss of approximately five pounds. The metabolic increase occurs within 10 minutes of drinking water.

4. Lose the sweet tooth

I know it's difficult for you sweet junkies to believe, but you can lose your desire for sweets. After following the Three Wisdoms program for several months, my patients find they no longer crave sweets and have better control of their appetite. If you can stick to the Three Wisdoms for three months, your entire attitude and feelings for food will change.

5. Treat the energy problem

If you've followed the **Nutrition-1-2-3** diet for a month and find you cannot lose weight or your energy has not picked up, then you may have an energy problem that is sabotaging your efforts. If you're anemic, have a thyroid imbalance or other health problem that is dragging you down, have it diagnosed and fixed. The help of a naturopathic physician may set you on the path toward better body composition.

Weight loss in a nutshell

I hope I've gotten the message across. Excess weight is detrimental to your health. History and modern research show that **Regularly eating a Variety of Whole foods** guarantees you will improve your body composition and feel better.

Chapter 27

Immune System Wisdoms –

Sick of being sick?

Do you suffer through cold and flu seasons with more than your fair share of drips, sneezes, snuffles and feeling low?

Proper nutrition is critical for a healthy functioning immune system. Yes, bug-fighting white blood cells require vitamins and minerals. If you're coming down with a serious infectious illness - one that keeps you home from work - more than once a year, you may need to look at your diet. This includes respiratory, urinary tract, lung, sinus, skin and vaginal infections. Your immune system should have the nutrients it needs to fight off infections, and keep them from becoming recurrent.

Another question to ask is, "Are you having more infections than you used to?"

Jill: More sick, more often

I remember Jill, a bus driver, who said, "I used to have a cold about every three years, then every year, and in the past two years I've had at least four." After reviewing Jill's health history and diet, we decided that she probably had a deficiency of protein. She'd become a vegetarian several years before. Unfortunately, she was not a very good vegetarian.

After increasing her protein intake for a couple of months she stopped getting sick. Jill's story is an illustration of how diet can influence immunity. In her case it was low protein intake, but it could have been a deficiency of zinc, vitamin A, or some other nutrient.

How often antibiotics?

Another way to evaluate your immune system is to ask how often you take antibiotics. The answer should be "I can't remember the last time I needed to take antibiotics." (Or any other prescription medication, for that matter.)

There are, of course, other reasons besides poor diet for having frequent infections. You may have a compromised immune system for some other reason. Just being low in blood iron can make you more susceptible. Sometimes it's necessary to seek out medical attention to rule out health problems that can lead to frequent infections. However, don't overlook the role of diet in keeping bugs at bay.

Antibiotic deficient, or your immune system?

Ideally, you should never have a need for chemical antibiotics except under certain extreme situations. For most infections, your own innate immune system does a great job.

I've treated upper respiratory infections, sore throats, sinus infections, wound infections, pneumonia, vaginal infections and even chronic diabetic leg ulcers using natural therapies. Some of these had been unsuccessfully treated with antibiotics before the patient came to me.

Did you know that antibiotics actually suppress your immune system? Yes, they hinder your white blood cells ability to attack and destroy germs. Antibiotics also disrupt the normal flora of the digestive system. By killing "good" bacteria, they make it easier for bad organisms to move in and cause you chronic problems. I see this often with children that have been inappropriately prescribed an antibiotic for an ear infection. Once their digestive function is compromised by antibiotics, these poor kids become increasingly susceptible to ear and respiratory tract infections.

The Surgeon General of the United States and most medical associations agree that antibiotics are widely overused and are the cause of the alarming increase in antibiotic-resistant infections. If you're taking antibiotics more than once every few years ask yourself, "Why isn't my immune system doing a better job?" A place to start fortifying your immune system is with the Three Wisdom diet.

It's not your job

Don't dismiss infectious diseases as a consequence of your job or the fact that you have small children. Yes, teachers are exposed to more runny noses, but not all teachers get sick several times a year.

Patty - School teacher with sinus headaches

My patient, Patty, a second-grade teacher, thought there was nothing else she could do for her mind-numbing sinus infections than take antibiotics. This had been going on for years. "Sinus infections are part of my life. I can practically mark them on the calendar."

After changing her diet she told me, "What a relief to not miss a week or more of work every semester while I lie in bed with my head throbbing - even when I took antibiotics."

Patty's problem? All the sugary treats she was eating along with the kids. Sugar suppresses the ability of your white blood cells to do their work.

If you're sick of being sick, take a close look at your diet and consider switching to a diet rich in the nutrients essential for your immune system to function optimally. The Three Wisdoms will super-size your immune system.

Chapter 28

Fight the Real War on Drugs –

Prescription and non-prescription drugs?

A good reason to consider overhauling your diet is if you're taking any prescription or non-prescription drug on a regular basis.

Whatever your medication is for, you may very well benefit from a nutrition program. Most conditions that people take medications for can be reduced or eliminated by diet therapy. The list is too long, but even serious medical problems such as asthma, diabetes, high blood pressure, high cholesterol and heart irregularities have shown to respond to nutritional intervention. And chronic non-fatal diseases such as irritable bowel disease, arthritis and most skin conditions respond positively to nutritional intervention.

According to the *Journal of the American Medical Association* (Vol. 284, July 26, 2000), 106,000 people died in 1999 from the negative effects of medications. The article rated "iatrogenic" as the third leading cause of death in the U.S. Iatrogenic is defined as "induced in a patient by a physician's activity, manner, or therapy, especially as a complication of treatment." Other researchers have estimated that between 100,000 and 200,000 people die every year in the U.S. from complications of the medical industry.

Statistics for 2007 found that in Florida that year 946 people died from illegal drugs, while 2,002 died from prescription drugs.

Besides the death rate from medications, there is also the cost in emergency department visits, extra physician visits and hospitalizations. Those are very scary statistics when you consider that the public-service organization Medwatch estimates that only 1 percent of all serious drug reactions are reported to the FDA.

Another argument against the unnecessary use of man-made drugs is that they are not natural to the body. Yes, I know, "natural" is a much misused word. But I use it in a very simple way. To me natural means something that the body evolved to deal with. Did the liver of a hunter-gatherer need to detoxify Tylenol, Zoloft or any of the other thousands of drugs that have been cooked up in the last 100 years? Actually, 90 percent of prescription drugs are less than 50 years old. It took millions of years for the liver to develop the capacity to detoxify natural substances. Fifty years is nothing in evolutionary time and makes us part of a vast biochemical experiment led by the pharmaceutical industry.

I'm not saying to stop any medication that has been prescribed for you. Getting off should be done under your physician's guidance. However, the right diet can eliminate or reduce your need for medication. I know these are strong words but I, and most nutrition-oriented doctors, have seen it happen time and again.

Let's spend a few minutes discussing a couple of common drugs.

Adrenal steroids

Various steroid medications - ointments, inhalers and pills - are commonly prescribed. They are powerful anti-inflammatories that are sometimes necessary for short-term use to save a life. Asthmatic patients often use them to enable them to breathe freely.

However, they are all too often prescribed for minor conditions for which they are unnecessary. Most of the time when steroids are prescribed, nothing is done about the patient's long-term, underlying problems. The original problem is still present, but is now covered up by a medication the can lead to serious side complications.

Steroids have a number of side effects. They can cause the retention of water, depress the patient's immune system, and "shut down" the patient's own production of adrenal steroids - a life-threatening condition.

Steroids may keep you alive in the event of a serious acute crisis. In the long run, however, steroids seriously undermine the health of your immune and repair systems.

I always ask my patients to consider their own inflammatory system. Yes, you have one. It is an elaborate network of cells, hormones and chemicals that travel throughout your body to protect you from foreign invaders. The question I help my patients solve is: why isn't your own anti-inflammatory system working?

If you can supply your immune system with the nutrients it needs, you may be able to wean yourself off steroids. It is in your best long-range interests.

Some of the nutrients found in the Three Wisdoms diet that are known to help support your natural anti-inflammatory system are selenium, zinc, vitamin C, the B vitamins, essential fatty acids and protein. My favorite bad guy, sugar, increases inflammation, as do bad fats.

A Pill for Everything

There are dozens of non-life-threatening diseases for which patients are prescribed unnecessary medicines. If the pharmaceutical industry had their way, you would be taking a pill for everything - obesity, erectile dysfunction, eczema, acne, headache, asthma, back pain, anxiety, depression, acid stomach, constipation, diarrhea, fatigue, allergies, poor concentration, insomnia, etc.

Yet, all of these conditions, and most any other illness you can think of, are successfully treated with natural therapies.

In almost all cases, drugs only treat the symptoms. They ignore the deeper problem. As I've discussed above in the case of anti-inflammatories, these drugs often, over the long run, make the condition worse or create other health problems.

If you're taking a medicine for a non-life-threatening condition, think carefully about who you want to trust with your health. Are you better off with a chemical brought to you by the pharmacological industry? Or would you rather trust your health to foods that have been nourishing people for hundreds of thousands of years?

Most likely your health problem is a relatively new disease of the past 200 years and is a consequence of a modern lifestyle – not enough exercise, increasing environmental pollution and a nutrient-poor diet.

The alternative to needless suffering and laboratory medications is a change in diet. Moving away from the nutrient-poor Standard American Diet (SAD) to the fortifying advantage of the Three Wisdoms is a great way to start rebuilding your health and kicking the drug habit.

Chapter 29

Pain Wisdoms –

Listen to the message

Where do you hurt? If you're like most people, you suffer from some form of chronic pain. Prescriptions for pain medication rose 88 percent between 1997 and 2005, according to the Drug Enforcement Administration. More than 200,000 pounds of the most powerful pain killers – codeine, morphine, oxycodone, hydrocodone and meperidine – are sold each year. That's enough for every American to take 300 milligrams (and someone took my share). Is this amount of pain normal? Can diet make a difference?

There was something about Mary, and it hurt

Mary was only thirty-five. As she sat telling me about various health problems including asthma, premenstrual syndrome, and heartburn, she rubbed her hands. After she finished telling me about herself, I asked her, "Do you have trouble with your hands?" She shrugged and said, "Not too much. Both my parents have arthritis, so..." She shrugged again as if this was to become her fate also. "I just forgot to take my aspirin today." She had become so used to her fingers hurting and so convinced there was nothing that could be done that she didn't mention it to me until I asked.

Although Mary didn't come to see me about her arthritis, I hoped it would help to explain the connections between her asthma, premenstrual syndrome, heartburn and arthritis. Often when looking at patients wholistically you can see the connections between seemingly unrelated symptoms.

I explained to her that her daily intake of aspirin might very well be triggering the heartburn and aggravating her asthma. Also, aspirin, while taking away the immediate pain, interferes with a joints' ability to heal. Additionally, it is common to see people with asthma also have a stomach condition – this corollary is part of the ancient sciences of acupuncture and oriental medicine. The overriding theme of Mary's symptoms was that they were all related to inflammation; inflammation of the stomach, joints and lungs.

We talked about the fact that joints can often repair and that she could become pain-free, if she would make a few changes in her diet. The first step was to stop taking aspirin and chemical anti-inflammatories and to switch over to natural anti-inflammatories.

> *"Omega-3 oils, from fish, and antioxidants from vegetables are fantastic for reducing pain."*

Omega-3 oils, from fish, and antioxidants from vegetables are fantastic for reducing pain.

Getting off aspirin was critical to her future because it actually slows down the healing process. Also, by irritating the stomach and intestinal lining it causes a condition called "leaky gut syndrome" in which small cracks form in the intestinal walls allowing toxins to pass through the wall and into the blood stream where they are transported to joints. This process of leaky gut-induced arthritis is not something I made up. It has been documented by scientists and published in prestigious medical journals. Yet, in spite of the availability of this knowledge, patients are still encouraged by doctors to take aspirin and other anti-inflammatory drugs every day.

By the way, don't think you're avoiding ulcers and leaky gut syndrome by using buffered aspirin. Aspirin blocks prostaglandins (See Fats 101 and Fats 102), which reduces mucus production. It's that mucus that helps protect the gut lining. Less mucus means less protection and more bleeding.

The body's balancing act

Under ideal circumstances, the body contains a balance of chemicals – those that induce inflammation, pro-inflammatory, and those that reduce inflammation, anti-inflammatory.

The pro-inflammatory chemicals act to protect us from infection and tissue damage. When you scrape your elbow, these chemicals rush to the site and start the repair process. This causes redness, swelling and pain, the cardinal signs of inflammation. Think of them as the firefighters that rush into a fire, spray water and other chemicals, chop down walls and search out every burning ember.

> *"We live in a pro-inflammatory world. Because of poor diets, stress and various toxins, our bodies become overburdened with firefighters and lack carpenters."*

Once the healing process is well under way, anti-inflammatory chemicals move in to clean up the debris and restore normalcy. These are the carpenter chemicals that clean up after the fire crew. (For more on this, see the EPA oils section in Fats 101.)

Our modern lifestyle was central to Mary's problems. We live in a pro-inflammatory world. Because of poor diets, stress and various toxins, our bodies become overburdened with firefighters and lack carpenters. This abundance of pro-inflammatory chemicals creates a tendency for inflammatory conditions such as arthritis, asthma, allergies, heart disease, stroke, irritable bowel syndrome, and inflammatory skin conditions. This is great for aspirin sales, but deadly to the body.

Treating Mary's pain

Mary and I went on to talk about how the same imbalance in her estrogen that was causing her premenstrual syndrome was contributing to her arthritis. Experiments strongly implicate estrogen as part of an imbalance that causes arthritis in some individuals. This is one reason women are more prone to develop this crippling disease.

I also suggested to Mary that her food allergies were probably contributing to her arthritis and that the aspirin was making her allergies worse. I finished this part of our talk by pointing out that her current diet of refined foods and few vegetables was depriving her joints of the nutrients they needed for repair. I felt her estrogen imbalance would probably take care of itself as her diet improved so there was no need for the natural, estrogen-balancing herbs that I sometimes use.

Mary agreed to change her diet, start taking fish oil supplements, drink a tea that would heal the lining of her intestines, and eliminate her allergic foods. She was aware that these changes would involve time and effort, but she was willing to do anything to feel better.

We started with the basics –

Regularity, Variety and Wholeness

I cautioned her about not getting discouraged because the physical changes in arthritic joints take months, even years, to reverse. I know from experience that sometimes patients become discouraged when they don't instantly feel better.

They are accustomed to the "Pill" model; take a pill and feel better now and don't worry about the future.

However, on Mary's second visit a few weeks later, she already felt better. "I'm surprised," she said, "I didn't think I could function without aspirin." I noticed she wasn't rubbing her hands. "I must admit, the only time my fingers hurt is after I've eaten sugar." Her heartburn was better also.

Over the next several months Mary saw her PMS and heartburn symptoms disappear and her fingers return to the same pain-free dexterity that other thirty-five year-olds experience.

Mary was lucky. Some patients, because they have more joint damage and other health problems, take longer to heal. But I have known eighty-year olds who swear by the anti-inflammatory effects of the Three Wisdoms.

"Inheriting" arthritis

I see many patients who talk about their arthritis as being a done deal because one or both of their parents have it. They change their thinking after making a few dietary changes. Usually their joints become more flexible and they are able to reduce or eliminate their need for medications.

What most patients don't realize is that while inheriting their parent's genes they also inherited their family's eating habits. Most children tend to eat a similar diet to their parents. They grow up eating what their parents put before them. They keep eating these foods because they know how to prepare them, are familiar with them, and can rely on them to be comforting.

Unfortunately, while familiarity is comforting, it can also lead to painful joints or other supposedly inherited diseases. These patients are unaware that the diet that they didn't choose but "inherited" predisposes them to arthritis because it lacks certain nutrients or has an imbalance of nutrients.

Headaches made worse

Headaches account for about 10 million doctors' visits a year. Why all this head pain? The reasons are complex. A good massage and learning some relaxation techniques would probably cure three-quarters of the headaches.

I view most headaches as an excess of inflammation. Tension headaches happen because muscles are inflamed. Part of the complexity of migraines is inflammation of blood vessels.

I do not conclude from this that the answer to headaches is to take a synthetic anti-inflammatory medication. Headaches are not the result of a deficiency of Advil, or whatever the current new "breakthrough" drug happens to be. The answer is to find the cause and treat it.

The long-term consequences of anti-inflammatory medications turn out to be quite negative for the pain sufferer. These drugs lower serotonin levels in the brain. Serotonin is a neurotransmitter, a chemical that relays messages in nerves. It inhibits pain. Pain drugs set in motion a devastating cycle. The pain "medicine" lowers serotonin and increases pain sensitivity which increases the need for more and stronger drugs. Not a bad deal for the pharmaceutical companies, but horrible for the headache sufferer.

There are natural alternatives to synthetic chemicals. These natural compounds can actually reduce your pain without reducing your health. Natural anti-inflammatories include such simple things as omega-3 oils, vitamins C, E and D, lipoic acid and zinc which are all found in whole foods. Certain herbs such as ginger and turmeric also contain natural anti-inflammatories.

The Three Wisdoms reduce inflammation

The Three Wisdoms have been shown in scientific studies to reduce inflammation:

- **Regularity** helps balance insulin, glucagon, growth hormone, cortisol and other chemical messengers involved with the inflammatory process.

- **Variety and Wholeness** (fresh, organic and unprocessed) increase the intake of naturally-occurring anti-inflammatory agents in foods: anti-oxidants, vitamins, minerals and omega-3 oils.

- **Wholeness** (organic) reduces the exposure to environmental toxins that exacerbate inflammation. Whole foods also contain more inflammation-fighting nutrients.

When in pain, don't look in the medicine cabinet, but seek out a healthy diet.

Chapter 30

Skin Wisdoms – Skin is the window of the body

It's easy for doctors and patients to focus on one problem, especially the skin, and lose sight of the bigger health picture.

Jim: A typical eczema case

Jim is a good example of just how deep skin problems can go. He came to see me because his sperm count was low. He and his wife had been trying to have a baby for several years. Initially their MD had concentrated on her inability to conceive. Finally, just at the time they had been thinking of undertaking expensive fertility treatments, it was suggested that he have his sperm count checked. Of course, this should have been done much earlier, but as so often happens, the burden of infertility is placed on the wife. On the recommendation of another patient, he came to see me.

Jim was generally healthy. On physical examination I discovered a large patch of eczema on his back. "Oh, that," he said, "That's just my eczema." Knowing that eczema often indicates more than just dry skin, I questioned him further.

As a child Jim suffered through many years of dry, red

skin. "I always wore long-sleeve shirts when I was a kid to hide my arms. I liked the cold weather, because then I could wear gloves, too." Because of his embarrassment, he never went on dates.

Now, at twenty-five, Jim controlled his skin with cortisone-based creams. He knew enough to not use them all the time, but three or four times a year he used them heavily. "I'll be fine for several months, only small patches on my arms, and then it'll spread everywhere." Jim had figured out that stress often initiated an outbreak. School exams, a new job, a week of overtime at work, would unleash the irritation and redness. "I know it's going to happen, but there's nothing I can do about it. Even the cortisone doesn't work."

We discussed Jim's general health and his diet in detail. I also ran some tests on him. When all the information was in, I pointed out three weaknesses in his diet: little water intake, poor-quality oil, and deficient zinc stores. These three factors could easily explain his eczema.

At the end of my explanation he was skeptical. "That seems too simple. I've had this all my life!"

"Most eczema is simple," I said. "Sometimes it's more difficult to treat. You may not be digesting your fats, but I'm going to presume that since your weight is normal and you don't have any overt digestive symptom, that's not a problem. You could also have food allergies. They can cause eczema. But, I didn't see any obvious evidence for that when we discussed your diet. We may have to revisit these possibilities later, but for now let's concentrate on water, zinc and the quality of your oils."

He asked, "If I'm low in zinc, why don't I have eczema all the time?"

"You're not completely depleted of zinc, but marginally low. Stress, both physical and mental, 'uses up' zinc. So, while normally you have enough zinc to keep your skin at a barely normal level, stress depletes your zinc.

When your zinc drops to below normal levels, your skin flares up. Zinc deficiency is common, partly because agricultural soil is often depleted and partly because of the over-consumption of sugar and refined carbohydrates."

The plan for Jim was simple: Drink two quarts of spring or filtered water each day. Switch from corn oil to organic, extra-virgin olive oil and organic nut oils. Eat zinc-rich foods such as organic poultry, sea foods, whole grains and nuts. Stop foods that steal zinc such as alcohol, sugar and refined carbohydrates.

Jim's response to the Three Wisdoms was typical. His skin started improving quickly. He noticed it was less dry within a week. After two months his eczema had cleared. Three months later, after several stressful twelve-hour days at work, a small patch of eczema appeared on his back. This was probably due to the stress of long hours, which reduce zinc stores, and his falling back into poor dietary habits during the overtime. But,

> "Jim, like many patients, came in focused on one problem, in his case a low sperm count, while ignoring a low-standing indicator of poor health: dry skin. Nutritionally-oriented doctors witness these kinds of successes every day."

after four years of following the Three Wisdoms, he still hadn't had another occurrence even though his stress level had gone up with the birth of a baby girl. Zinc also affects fertility levels and was the determining factor in raising his sperm count.

Jim, like many patients, came in focused on one problem, in his case a low sperm count, while ignoring a low-standing indicator of poor health: dry skin. Nutritionally-oriented doctors witness these kinds of successes every day.

Skin and oil:
Eczema, acne and other skin problems

Under normal circumstances, skin produces oils that lubricate and protect it. If there is a problem with the oil - too much, too little, the wrong kind, or bacterial contamination - skin conditions result.

I tell my patients that the quality of their skin's oils depends on these things:

- The type of oils eaten.
- Your ability to digest and process the oil adequately.
- Food allergies.
- Your supply of vitamin and mineral cofactors - especially vitamins A and E, and zinc.
- Other dietary factors also have a positive influence on the skin. Fiber, for instance, improves digestive function and slows the release of sugars, which reduces the incidence of acne. Excessive intake of sugar increases glucose levels in the skin which promotes the growth of acne-causing bacteria.
- Water helps the skin by providing hydration and helping the kidneys and bowels eliminate wastes.

The **Nutrition-1-2-3** program provides the necessary nutrients, aids digestion and reduces the intake of sweets. It also provides high-quality oils that eventually make their way into the skin.

Always look below the surface

Skin conditions are medical problems that, while usually not life threatening, are "indicator" diseases. They act as a barometer of a person's general health.

It's not unusual for a patient to come in with a host of other problems and not even mention their scaly, dry skin, acne, or other chronic problems. Sadly, they've been taught that their skin condition is not treatable except with cortisone and other creams.

Many skin problems, even life-long chronic ones, respond well to the Three Wisdoms. If your skin doesn't improve after three months, there is probably another problem. Speak with a doctor who understands the importance of good digestion and the impact of food sensitivities on health.

Chapter 31

Cancer Wisdoms –
Let's stop losing the war on cancer

Cancer is an enormous and complicated subject so I'd like to just mention a few things about it in relation to diet.

Family History

Do you have a strong family history of cancer? If so, don't discount that history, but also don't despair. While cancer is partially influenced by genetics, environmental toxins and diet are at least a fifty percent influence. Some authors state that environment accounts for eighty percent of cancer incidence.

Ideally, a strong family history of cancer will inspire you to not give up on yourself, but to go on a cancer-prevention program.

Because there are many types of cancer, not all cancer-prevention programs are the same. However, I would argue that the foundation of any cancer-defense program is a top-notch diet – the Three Wisdoms program.

Your body is working to stop cancer every second of the day. You have various internal processes for weeding out cancer-causing chemicals and also for policing abnormal cell growth. Think about the energy and nutrients required for this constant surveillance system. It requires a 24/7 work schedule to recognize and kill or expel cancer-causing chemicals and early cancer cells. We don't fully understand all there is to know about the body's innate cancer-screening systems, but what we do know is that these processes require protein, essential fatty acids, vitamins, and minerals.

Research priorities

Thousands of scientists and millions of dollars are being devoted to finding a cure for cancer. Unfortunately, only a very small percentage of that research involves diet and lifestyle. In the research community the study of diet is not as sexy or lucrative as drugs. Most research money flows toward new therapies that can be patented. Patents mean exclusive ownership. And patents mean money. Lots of money.

Since 1971 and the beginning of the War on Cancer, many billions of dollars have been spent on this battle. While hopes have been raised with every new "miracle" drug, none has lived up to the title. You've read about it, the "breakthrough" that will change cancer treatment, but you've forgotten the name because it quickly fell from the headlines.

Meanwhile, currently one in eight women develops breast cancer compared to one in twenty of their mothers.

With all the billions of dollars and thousands of research hours, no unified theory on cancer has resulted. No widely-applicable therapy has been developed. Fifteen hundred Americans die each day from the devastating effects of cancer. One in every three American women and one in two men develop a malignancy. Yet the money keeps flowing from your pocket, through the IRS, with decrees by Congress, to private and university-based research programs looking for drugs.

When nutrition studies are funded, most have to do

with using a specific, individual nutrient. Not surprisingly, these nutrients are either owned through patents or controlled by one corporation because of the complexities of manufacturing. If a corporation is the sole or principal manufacturer of a vitamin, then it is in its interest to encourage studies that measure the effectiveness of that nutrient in cancer.

Where is the "magic bullet"?

It is true that studying drugs and individual nutrients is much easier and far less expensive than funding research on general nutrition. This narrow hunt is also a bias for most researchers. Too many of them are looking for the "magic bullet", the single product that will cure cancer. Too few researchers will admit what they all know to be true; cancer is not a single disease. There are multiple chemical, hormonal and immunological processes that take part in the development of cancer and therefore no single agent will cure all forms of cancer.

The "magic bullet" approach is counter to how the body works. Cancer, like most diseases, is the outcome of a multitude of interactions: between chemistry and function, between the external environment and the inside of the body, and between the many aspects of nutrition and the functioning of all organs.

In spite of the concentration of cancer research on drugs and single synthetic vitamins, over 128 scientific studies have shown that eating fruits and vegetables protects against cancers. We also know that certain nutrients enhance the liver's ability to detoxify cancer-inducing chemicals. Wouldn't you like to eat more of these protective nutrients? You can by Regularly eating a Variety of Whole foods.

I bring up the failures of cancer research not to say that the National Institute of Cancer (NIC) should be disbanded, but to point out the complexities and difficulties it faces. My criticism is that they are stuck in the old "magic bullet" approach and are often blind to a whole-system, panoramic view of the problem. They are also too locked into the drug industry and are not able or willing to look to the wisdom of the body and the value of enhancing natural processes with natural compounds.

Most of all, I do not believe that the scarcity of nutritional studies should prevent you from doing the best you can to prevent cancer by applying good nutrition. Although cancer screening and early treatment has improved, some forms of cancer are on the rise. There is good evidence that the modern industrial diet that is high in calories, pesticides and other chemicals, and low in nutrients is part of the cancer problem.

The **Nutrition-1-2-3** diet reduces your risk of cancer by decreasing your exposure to toxic chemicals and providing you with a rich supply of the nutrients your own internal anti-cancer system needs to do its work.

Diagnoses of Cancer

What if you've already been diagnosed with cancer?

I am not claiming that diet alone will cure your cancer, but it is often the people who have incorporated a healthy diet that achieve victory, even in severe cases. Naturally, you want to include other lifestyle changes such as stress reduction, meditation and exercise, to maximize your body's healing potential.

In addition, there are some promising scientific reports showing the benefit of a nutritious diet in battling cancer. Of course, much more research needs to be done. Unfortunately, while there is plenty of money to research drugs that can be patented, there is little money for investigating vegetables. In the meantime, however, you are helping yourself if you eat the best diet possible during your journey to regain your health.

Even if changing your diet doesn't cure your cancer, it

will strengthen your immune system and reduce the load of cancer-causing chemicals on your body. If you need chemotherapy, surgery or radiation, it will help you to be in the best condition you can be before starting.

Also, even if you are already undergoing therapy for cancer, a healthy intake of vitamins and minerals may help decrease the side effects of the therapy, which is often quite toxic. And a good diet will benefit you during your recovery stage.

A number of natural antioxidants including vitamins A, D and E, zinc, selenium and flavonoids have shown promise against different types of cancers. A Variety of Whole foods are rich in antioxidants. Ditto adequate protein and healthy oils. They help your body keep fit. Nutrition can make a significant difference.

Consult with your cancer specialist before embarking on any diet change, but the Three Wisdoms program is not radical and should not alarm any doctor that understands basic nutritional concepts.

Beans against cancer

I love this research study because it illustrates the power of diet using one of the least sexy foods: beans.

Most of us know more about the latest "breakthrough" treatment for cancer. You might have read how venture capital is backing a new biotech company with a "promising" new drug.

However, you probably missed the research coming out of the Department of Agriculture's Bean Research Unit. What, you missed that on the nightly news?

It turns out those beans are rich in antioxidants and fiber and are strongly related to a decrease in cancer cases.

Surely your doctor mentioned that the World Health Organization recommends you eat one ounce of beans four times a week because that intake level has been shown to lower your cancer risk by twenty-two percent? Try finding a million-dollar drug that can do as well.

Studies have found that cheap, non-patented, and non-genetically engineered beans can lower rates of breast, prostate and colon cancers. One researcher (Hangen 2002) found that beans reduced the incidence of colon cancer by over fifty percent!

Population studies show that countries where the people consume more beans, such as in Mexico, have much lower rates of colon, rectal, breast and prostate cancers than countries such as Poland, Czech Republic and Slovenia, where the populations consume few beans.

So what'll you have, the latest, greatest chemical treatment, or a bowl of beans?

Even the American Cancer Society watches diet

When I started my medical practice in the early 1980s, the American Cancer Society's (ACS) stand was that diet had no effect on cancer. To their credit, they've started paying attention to the research and now encourage people to eat broccoli and other vegetables that have shown positive results against cancer.

When a conservative, drug-oriented institution like the ACS comes out in favor of nutrition, the research must be overwhelming. Time and again studies have concluded that some of the best defenses against cancer are real vegetables, avoiding excessive calories, and eating a variety of foods. Sound familiar? Do I need to repeat the Three Wisdoms?

Chapter 32

Sugar Wisdoms – Diabetes, hypoglycemia and sugar diseases

The not-so-sweet epidemic

Adult-onset diabetes and hypoglycemia, the most common blood sugar disorders, kill and debilitate millions of people every year. Diabetes is high blood sugar while hypoglycemia means low blood sugar. They are both newly emerging diseases, having sprung forth in the last two hundred years because of the sorry state of our diets.

Diabetes

Adult onset or Type 2 diabetes is dramatically increasing in the United States. As of 2005, 18.2 million people have been diagnosed with diabetes which is about 6.3% of the population. Trillions of dollars are being spent on treatment.

Even sadder, children are increasingly affected. While twenty years ago only about two percent of the new cases of diabetes were in 9 to 19 year old children, now it's thirty to fifty percent. Many experts say that the vast majority of child diabetics are not diagnosed. Instead they are labeled as "slow learners" and "behavioral problems."

In the next 25 years, the death rate from diabetes is estimated to go from 16 to 50 million persons per year. It is already the sixth leading cause of death in the U.S. These numbers are particularly frightening when you realize that an estimated twenty-five percent of cases go undiagnosed.

The long-term health consequences of diabetes are not slight. It is a leading cause of obesity, heart disease, cancer, kidney dysfunction, blindness and circulatory problems.

Hundreds of billions of dollars are being spent on the treatment of diabetes and its complications. With the numbers of aging baby boomers, estimates are that soon several trillion dollars will go into diabetes treatment each year.

> "Diabetes is a horrible and crippling disease that can kill. However, you can fight back. Its two main enemies are exercise and diet."

All this money, misery and death are unnecessary. Type 2 Diabetes is a preventable disease. Results of the Nurses Health Study, which has been in progress for 17 years, have shown a 90 percent decrease in adult onset, Type 2, diabetes among participants leading a healthy lifestyle. That lifestyle included keeping weight down, eating a high-fiber diet with low levels of trans-fatty acids, and regular exercise; nothing radical and no drugs.

Numerous studies have demonstrated how something as simple as eating whole grains can improve glucose regulation. (See *American Journal of Clinical Nutrition* 2001; 75.848-855.)

Diabetes is a horrible and crippling disease that can kill. However, you can fight back. Its two main enemies are exercise and diet. It's a terrible waste to be spending trillions of dollars on palliative diabetes care when that money could be used to improve schools or to provide healthcare for those without.

The **Nutrition-1-2-3** program is far more important than your genetic inheritance – no matter how many relatives you have with diabetes. Follow the Three Wisdoms way and watch your risk for developing diabetes drop.

Hypoglycemia

Hypoglycemia is defined as low blood sugar and it's a common problem in American society. The patient often has a blood sugar that "roller coasters" up and down throughout the day. Insulin, glucagon and other hormone levels also follow a similar unstable pattern. It results in fatigue, mental confusion, headaches, irritability, forgetfulness, depression and anxiety, to name a few symptoms.

Diagnosis can be made through a qualified physician. Generally people can figure out they have hypoglycemia if they experience any of the above symptoms 2 to 4 hours after eating a high-carbohydrate meal or snack.

If you suffer from hypoglycemia, the Three Wisdoms can make a profound difference in your life. Just doing one of them - eating regularly - can work wonders for many sufferers.

Sugar Diseases

There are a number of diseases that are associated with sugar and refined carbohydrate consumption. Entire books have been written on this subject.

A list of diseases associated with sugar and refined carbohydrate consumption includes: hypoglycemia, diabetes, obesity, metabolic syndrome (a combination of obesity, diabetes, hypertension and high blood fats), diverticulitis, irritable bowel syndrome, gallstones, peptic ulcers, varicose veins, hemorrhoids, acne, frequent infections, pre-menstrual syndrome, cancer, macular degeneration, depression, cardiovascular disease, hypertension, cataracts, learning disabilities, neuropathy, infertility and chronic fatigue.

This list might sound like an exaggeration. How could eating sugar be associated with so many health problems? These conditions are all linked to deficiencies of certain vitamins and minerals that are "stolen" by the consumption of sugar. Also, sugar throws off the body's balance of insulin and glucagon and increases inflammation in the body. And, just to add more insult to injury, conditions like diverticulitis, gallstones, varicose veins and hemorrhoids are all associated with the lack of fiber as found in refined carbohydrates.

Sugar kills and debilitates millions of people each year. The medical literature is very clear on this. And it's no secret that the problem is getting worse.

No matter how much money is spent on high-tech research and development for diabetic drugs, the problem will not get any better until the underlying cause is addressed. You must stop eating refined sugar.

Adult-onset or Type 2 diabetes is nearing epidemic proportions among baby boomers. Diabetes is the sixth leading cause of death in the U.S. (2008). It once struck only one in fifty thousand Americans. Now it strikes one in twenty. Some experts feel that this one condition could, over the next two decades, bankrupt our healthcare system.

Forms of diabetes: Juvenile vs. Adult

When most people think about diabetes they assume it's a genetic disease. There are two forms of diabetes: juvenile (Type 1) and adult-onset (Type 2). Juvenile diabetes accounts for about 5 to 10 percent of cases. This type has a strong genetic association. Adult-onset diabetes makes up the vast majority of cases and is a result of life-style factors such as diet and exercise.

A more descriptive name for adult-onset diabetes is insulin-resistant diabetes. (For a review of sugar and insulin, see Chapter 6, Carbohydrates 101.) In this type of diabetes, cells literally become more resistant to insulin because they are bombarded with excessive amounts of dietary sugar. This unnatural bombardment "wears out" the cell and makes insulin less effective. The cell becomes unable to obey insulin's signal to transport glucose into the cell. The continuing high blood glucose levels trigger signals for higher and higher insulin output from the pancreas. As the body keeps secreting more insulin, the cells become more resistant. Without the effect of the insulin, blood sugar levels go up while intercellular levels go down. Thus, the cell starves and the blood sugar levels climb. Eventually the patient is diagnosed with diabetes.

Juvenile, or type 1, diabetes is now believed to be a partially a genetic disease. The theory is that a genetic weakness becomes triggered by a virus. In this type of diabetes, diet is a mainstay of therapy, along with the use of insulin injections. The goal of nutrition here is to consume a Regular balance of protein, fats and carbohydrates with the goal of decreasing glucose swings.

Cure for the sweet tooth

If you describe yourself as having a "sweet tooth" or feel victimized by a sugar addiction, the best place to start your return to health is with the Three Wisdoms.

Regularity, Variety and Wholeness help balance blood sugar, insulin and other hormone levels.

One example of how Wholeness helps blood sugar control is that it supplies generous amounts of fiber. Fiber is known to slow the absorption of glucose from the digestive system into the blood stream. This alone reduces the fast influx of glucose into the blood and the resulting high insulin response.

Another benefit of eating whole foods is that they provide low saturated fats and high omega-3 fats. This creates a change in cell membranes that makes them more sensitive to insulin signaling.

The **Nutrition-1-2-3** diet will help you control your blood sugar. It has helped diabetics discontinue their medications. This is not something I claim lightly. There are literally millions of Type 2, adult-onset diabetics who could easily do away with their oral diabetic medications if they would make a few changes in their lifestyle. This has been proven in multiple experiments.

Additionally, we know that the high vitamin and mineral content of whole foods reduces blood sugar levels and the complications of diabetes.

Please, if you have a "sweet tooth", don't continue down the road of least resistance. Fight back against the drug sugar and save yourself from needless suffering.

Rant against eating sugar

Sugar offers no environmental, medical or health benefits. It is, instead, a detriment to the land, society and personal health. The negative impact of sugar has been known for at least 200 years and is well-established by current scientific research. All individuals who care about the health of the planet and their personal well-being should avoid it.

Given sugar's enormous cost to society, efforts should be made to increase taxes on it, such as tobacco and alcohol are taxed. I would argue that the connection between sugar and diabetes is so strong that a case can be made for a class-action suit against the sugar industry. Just as the tobacco companies have been shown to be liable and made to pay for smoking-related deaths, big sugar should pay for the sugar diseases - diabetes being the worst, but not the only, of many health problems related to sugar.

It's the diet

The real tragedy is that Type 2 diabetes and hypoglycemia are usually entirely preventable with simple lifestyle changes and without the use of medications. Even Type 1 patients could reduce their vulnerability to the devastating complications of this disease.

The effectiveness of diet in preventing and treating diabetes is not a carefully guarded secret. Since diabetes was first discovered, doctors have been aware that sugar consumption made the condition worse. In the past, they diagnosed it by tasting the sweetness of the patient's urine. Unfortunately this basic lesson has been lost to most contemporary MD's who, amazingly, regard sugar as a food even thought it is well established as an anti-food.

There are also numerous historic lessons that teach us about the relationship between diet and diabetes. For instance, during World War I, the incidence of diabetes decreased drastically when sugar was rationed.

Laboratory experiments and epidemiologic studies also support the connection between diet (especially the intake of sugar) and blood sugar problems.

If you have hypoglycemia or diabetes, you need to change your diet. Three simple words - Regularity, Variety and Wholeness - can save your life.

Chapter 33

Heart Wisdoms – High cholesterol and blood pressure

Carl: the heart of the matter

"I feel like I have no choice." Carl, a Boeing engineer, sat in my office holding out four bottles of prescription medicine. "They tell me I have to take these for the rest of my life."

Carl's story is not unusual. His blood pressure and cholesterol had been steadily rising for ten years; so had his weight. His MD started prescribing pills early on because of Carl's strong family history of heart disease. By fifty Carl felt like an old man. He had been through a series of different medicines because after a year or two they would stop working. When he came in to see me he felt prescription pills were his only option, yet even with them he still had borderline high blood pressure and cholesterol readings.

Carl said, "I know I have to take these pills. I have this family history. But, do I have to feel so worn out all the time?"

I explained to Carl that his low energy and heart problems were related. His cholesterol, blood pressure and weight were going up for the same reasons his energy was low. The body works as a whole, integrated organism. When you stress one part of it, you inevitably stress other areas. When your energy is low, you don't burn calories, break down cholesterol and lose fat like you should. The extra weight and stress on the body forces the heart to work harder. Vessels become hardened and more pressure must be used to pump the blood. There are many complex chemical and mechanical interactions all intersecting to create the deadly situation in which Carl found himself.

I pointed out that while Carl did have the same genes as his parents, his more important inheritance was his style of eating. He was consuming the same high-starch diet of his parents and grandparents, but he wasn't working long hours on a farm like they had. He was sitting at a desk.

To make matters worse, the starches he was eating were not the whole-grain and organic vegetables his grandparents ate, but the highly-refined, nutrient-poor, and pesticide-laden foods of modern America.

While genes are a factor in heart disease, in most cases they're much less of a problem than lifestyle.

When I explained to Carl the principles of **Nutrition-1-2-3** he said, "Why didn't my MD ever explain how simple it was? I thought I'd have to eat one of those macrobiotic diets and never eat beef, cheese and all the foods I like."

When Carl came back to see me a month later he admitted that, while the Three Wisdoms are easy to understand, "It was a big change for a meat, bread and donut guy like myself." Nevertheless, even by just eating a small protein-rich breakfast and cutting his sugar intake by about a third, he felt better.

Carl progressed like many patients. The more he followed the program, the better he felt. The better he felt, the more he adhered to the program. Within six months he'd lost twenty pounds, his blood pressure was normal and, with the cooperation of his MD, he was beginning to reduce his medications.

"Best of all," he told me, "I've got a life after work. I'm even thinking about taking up your suggestion to exercise." We both laughed at that.

By the end of a year, Carl had transformed himself from having a vertical disease and living among the ranks of the walking wounded, into a well man, free of potentially harmful drugs, with a healthy cardiovascular system, and enough energy to live a fulfilling life. While not a star athlete, he's gotten quite fond of taking long bike rides several days a week.

If you have heart disease, food can be your worst enemy or best friend. It's your choice. Give healthy eating a chance to become your friend.

Bill: We all have a choice

"Do I really need to be taking this pill? I'm only thirty. I'm healthy." Bill had another typical story. Unlike Carl, he had no family history of heart disease and no other risk factors. He was even enthusiastic about doing whatever changes seemed necessary to bring down his cholesterol. But his MD had never considered any of these factors. One borderline-high cholesterol reading had, in his MD's opinion, earned Bill a prescription for a drug of questionable benefit and potential danger.

A person who has high cholesterol, high blood pressure, a family history of heart disease and other blood indicators of increased risks of cardiac problems such as high uric acid, homocysteine, triglycerides and C-reactive protein, may feel that the risk of taking cholesterol-lowering statin drugs is worth it. Most people, however, can reduce all of these risk factors with simple dietary changes.

The Three Wisdoms have been shown to reduce all of the risk factors associated with heart disease. Regularity reduces obesity and cholesterol. Variety increases antioxidants. Whole foods reduce exposure to chemicals known to damage blood vessels and increase vital nutrients.

Some MDs argue that most people will not make the necessary dietary changes to reduce cholesterol. I hear the opposite from my patients. They're willing to make changes, but are often confused as to the best course to follow. Media reports confuse them. Fad diets seem too extreme. Their MDs' only advice is written on a prescription pad. What most patients hear, from the media and the medical community, is a confusion of half-facts and bad advice. It's no wonder they give up and take the pills.

Wrong prescription. Wrong advice.

The media and medical community are fixated on the idea that eating less fat is the diet solution to high cholesterol. This notion has been a fixture in the U.S. for almost half a century. Low-fat foods are a huge industry. People who know nothing else about diet will read labels to find out how much fat is lurking in their TV dinner, oblivious to the fact that their low-fat menu choice has little protein, fiber or other nutrients.

The food industry has even taken natural products such as milk and de-fattened them, even though whole milk is already relatively low in fat with only 3 to 6 percent.

Is fat the problem?

The common wisdom seems to be that eating cholesterol increases blood cholesterol. However, look at what the statistics show. In the past 20-plus years, the U.S. population has lowered its fat intake by 14 percent and increased its sugar and carbohydrate percentage by 110 percent and cholesterol levels have continued to rise. Cholesterol-lowering drugs have flourished along with the low-fat diet foods.

An interesting fat question is: If fats are so bad for you, why is it that multiple studies have shown that eating nuts, which are one of the highest-fat foods in nature, actually lowers blood lipids and increases the good HDL fats?

The answer is simply that: Quality matters more than quantity.

Natural, high-quality fats are good for you. Nuts (non-roasted, un-salted and otherwise un-corrupted) were eaten by hunter-gatherers. The types of fats that the average American eats today including soy, corn and trans-fats are not "natural" and were not eaten by our hereditary ancestors. (See Chapters 9 & 10: Fats 101 and 102 for more details.)

There are certainly people who eat too much fat. Far more people, however, eat too much starch and not enough fiber, which are the two most common reasons for having high blood fat (and weight gain).

The fact that the liver manufactures cholesterol and that cholesterol is necessary for life (because many hormones are manufactured from it) and that our pre-historic ancestors ate much more of it than we do is not conveyed to most patients.

Too few patients are given helpful information about the functions of cholesterol or about useful dietary information of any kind. More often, a busy hand quickly writes a prescription and, having writ, moves on.

High Blood Pressure

Re-read the above sections and substitute the words "cholesterol-lowering drugs" with "blood-pressure lowering drugs". The same principles apply and the same diet solutions work. Research has proven it multiple times.

Yes, there is a small percentage of people who probably benefit from taking blood-pressure lowering drugs. On the other hand, many more people have them prescribed when they would do much better with a few simple alterations in their diet and lifestyle.

A natural diet as described in **Nutrition-1-2-3** is full of blood-pressure lowering vitamins, minerals and other food factors. One example is magnesium, shown in numerous studies to be commonly deficient in industrial-society diets. Magnesium naturally lowers blood pressure. Omega-3 oils and fiber do the same.

What is malpractice?

I submit that most of the prescriptions written for cholesterol and blood pressure-lowering drugs are done so out of haste, laziness and ignorance. What has happened to the part of the Hippocratic Oath that says, "First, do no harm."?

Presently, cholesterol and blood pressure-lowering drugs are among the most commonly prescribed medications in the U.S. They are handed out like candy, usually with little or no counseling as to the side effects or alternatives. A brief list of a much

> Numerous studies have shown that simple lifestyle changes can effectively lower cholesterol.

longer inventory of known side-effects includes muscle wasting, electrolyte imbalances, vitamin and mineral depletion, cancer, fatigue, and increased incidence of suicide.

According to the AMA, prescription drugs account for over 100,000 deaths each year in the U.S. That makes them the fourth leading cause of death. Shouldn't that alert the medical community to take a long hard look at their style of practice? But, it's a rare MD who takes the time to explain the side-effects, limitations or alternatives to prescription medicines.

Do the benefits of these drugs outweigh their potential for harm? No one knows. There are no long-term studies that show that cholesterol-lowering drugs prolong life or are free of serious side effects. Some studies have found that while they lower cholesterol, they also increase overall death rates. Few patients are told this.

Are there safer alternatives? Yes. Numerous studies

have shown that simple lifestyle changes can effectively lower cholesterol. And I do mean simple. For most people their cholesterol can be lowered without the need for major life or diet changes.

Is the alternative difficult?

I believe that most patients would have the good sense to stay away from cholesterol and blood pressure medications if they understood (1) the minimal known benefits, (2) the potential risks and (3) how easy the alternatives are to incorporate.

To cite one study: The prestigious *New England Journal of Medicine* (1999) found that eating a small portion of fiber, in the form of oatmeal, lowered cholesterol by 30 percent. The editors commented that this was the equivalent to taking a cholesterol-lowering drug.

How difficult is it to give this information to a patient? Judging by the number of prescriptions written, most MDs find this too time consuming, tedious or beyond their scope of knowledge.

There may be patients who are unable to lower their cholesterol by increasing their fiber. For them there are other alternatives such as the complete Three Wisdoms program. There are also vitamins and other natural food supplements that can return cholesterol to normal.

Blood pressure and cholesterol-lowering drugs, like all drugs, should be reserved for patients who have not responded to non-drug intervention and who are at clear risk of heart disease.

How the Three Wisdoms save your heart

This diet contains all of the elements that have been shown by researchers to protect against hardening of the arteries, high blood pressure, elevated cholesterol, increased clotting and inflammation.

1. High fiber

Lowers cholesterol and helps control blood sugar (another risk factor).

2. High levels of vitamins and minerals.

Especially vitamin E, magnesium, potassium and zinc from whole grains, fruits and vegetables.

3. High levels of omega-3 oils.

From fish, organic meats and vegetables. Reduces inflammation and clotting.

4. Reduces inflammation in the vessels.

Cholesterol is deposited where there is inflammation.

5. Reduces homocysteine.

Homocysteine is a chemical found in the blood of everyone. Too much is an independent risk factor for heart disease that is decreased by certain B-vitamins found in whole grains.

6. Reduces blood pressure.

Because of high levels of several factors including magnesium, potassium and B-vitamins, while being low in sodium.

7. Reduces cholesterol.

Because it is low in refined carbohydrates and bad fats and high in fiber.

8. Reduces LDL (bad) cholesterol.

People only eating one meal daily had large increases in LDL cholesterol according to a study by the USDA and National institute on Aging. Another good reason for Regular meals and snacks.

9. Eliminates hydrogenated oils.

These damage vessels and reduce the ability of nutrients to pass into the cell.

10. Lowers weight.

Excess weight is a known factor in increasing heart disease risk.

11. High in anti-oxidants.

Anti-oxidants such as vitamins C and E protect the heart from the damaging effects of bad fats. (*Journal of the American Medical Association*, Nov. 1997).

Treat the New Disease with Ancient Foods

Heart and vascular diseases are new. They were first described in the medical literature in 1910. The reason they are the number-one killer in Western societies is because of the Western lifestyle, especially the refined food diet.

Your best weapon against cardiovascular disease is to return to the diet that protected people from heart disease for thousands of years. Regularity, Variety and Wholeness describe the ancient diet.

All one heart

The heart and blood vessels (cardiovascular system) are very responsive to nutritional imbalances. They work continuously, twenty-four hours a day, and require a great deal of energy and repair nutrients. Just like your car engine will go more miles if it is given the best fuel and lubricants, so too will your heart and vessels. **Nutrition-1-2-3** will help insure your heart receives the nutrition it needs to keep you away from the drugstore.

Chapter 34

Breathing Wisdoms - Asthma and respiratory diseases

Shelly: I just want to breathe normally

"My MD exploded when I told him I was thinking of coming to see you." Shelly, a slender, smiling woman in her 30s, confessed to me. "He told me if I tried naturopathic treatments I'd end up in the emergency room. I just want to breathe normally, without an inhaler."

Sally had suffered from asthma since she was a child. In her 20s she'd been hospitalized several times with dangerous breathing difficulty. She knew first hand the horrible feeling of not getting enough oxygen into her lungs. It was very brave of her to look for answers outside the medical-industrial system.

The first thing I did was explain to Shelly the mechanism of inflammation in asthma and that she would feel better when the inflammation was reduced. I also advised her, "Use your inhaler like you always have - when you need it. I think you will find that you'll need it less and less."

Shelly returned after being on the Three Wisdoms program for two weeks. "I haven't used my inhaler in two days. I know it seems crazy, but I can feel air moving into parts of my lungs that have been closed down for years."

It's been several years since I first met Shelly and she now uses her inhaler only rarely. She has found that the most important parts of the diet for her are avoiding sweets and rotating her foods so that she avoids the ones she's sensitive to because they increase inflammation and aggravate her breathing.

Her MD's warning, while well-intentioned, was alarmist and based on no evidence. Real-world experiences show that it is the patients who exclusively use prescription asthma medications who are ending up in emergency rooms. Each year more patients who only use drugs and only treat the symptoms end up hospitalized and each year more die. If I was an alarmist I would tell her that asthma medications kill.

What is asthma?

In the simplest terms, asthma is an inflammation of the lungs that causes the air spaces to constrict. This creates a restricted flow of oxygen. It is possible for the restriction to be so mild that the person is not aware of it. Their only symptom might be a degree of fatigue. At the other extreme, the breathing may become so restricted that the patient cannot get in enough oxygen to stay alive.

Most of us understand inflammation. It's part of what happens if you sprain an ankle or cut yourself. It is also part of the symptoms you experience with a cold. In the case of asthma, your lungs exhibit the classic signs of inflammation - heat, swelling, and redness. Unlike the twisted ankle, you can't see your lungs, but you can feel the results of the inflammation.

Inflammation is a natural part of the body's defense system. The symptoms you experience result from your body trying to heal itself.

In asthma, the lungs are inflamed because something irritates and causes them to react or even to over-react. The over-reaction triggers swelling of the tissues and spasms in the muscles. There becomes, literally, less space for oxygen.

When you know the mechanism of asthma, certain treatment options become obvious. First, remove the irritant. Second, stop the lungs from becoming inflamed.

Treating asthma and lung inflammation

Environmental treatment

It is no coincidence that lung problems are getting worse as the air we breathe becomes less breathable. Billions of tons of poisons of various kinds are pumped into the environment by factories that, for the most part, are producing consumer goods and useless paraphernalia that soon end up in landfills and incinerators. The military with its chemical weapons, jet airplanes and radiation hazards are huge polluters of the environment.

The medical industry, while trying to create its drug "miracles," generates millions of tons of lung-inflaming contaminants. Drug manufacturing and packaging require solvents, acids, dyes, chemical reactants, radioactive isotopes, and a host of other environmentally unfriendly substances. When the day is done, as someone stands in front of a shelf of two dozen remedies for their sore throat, the chemicals used to manufacture, package and ship that drug are floating in our streams, piled into our land fills, and suspended in our air.

Adding insult to injury, some over-the-counter drugs, such as acetaminophen (Tylenol), actually increase the risk of asthma. (Thorax, 2000 and *European Respiratory Journal*, 2000, to name two references.)

To make matters worse, while we blithely contaminate the air, we cut down the forests which are the recycling system for renewing our oxygen supply.

A basic step toward eradicating asthma would be to start cleaning up the air. **Nutrition-1-2-3** contributes to a cleaner environment by emphasizing the use of organic foods that are not processed, overly-packaged or shipped long distances. By eating fresh, healthy foods that are grown close to home, you contribute to the fight against land, water and air pollution.

Individual treatment

The person with asthma will benefit from avoiding things that trigger an attack. Breathing clean fresh air, when available, helps. Home air cleaners are also of great benefit. Don't just buy what is heavily advertised or looks hip and cool. Read Consumer Reports for their periodic evaluation of home air cleaning systems. According to past reports, some of the most popular units are the least effective.

Allergies, salt, food additives, and preservatives, particularly sulfites, are all known to increase the severity and frequency of asthmatic attacks.

A Variety of organic foods are rich in nutrients which have been found to help asthmatics especially vitamins B-6, B-12, and C, magnesium, molybdenum and selenium. Omega-3 oils from oily fish are also known to lessen the symptoms of asthma.

Dietary micronutrients such as flavonoids and antioxidants, which are emphasized in the Three Wisdoms diet, are also beneficial. I have seen many patients just like Shelly stop using their asthma medications after following the Three Wisdoms.

Both traditional Chinese medicine and natural Western medicine link asthma to digestive system problems. Whole foods with plenty of fiber and water help support digestion and elimination.

Asthma is a serious and sometimes deadly disease. I'm not recommending anyone throw their asthma prescription away. I'm saying that most people will feel better and have less of a need for their medication after one to six months of following the Three Wisdoms. In fact, I've seen patients feel better in just days. It's perfectly safe to follow a healthy diet of whole foods along with your medicine.

"Miracle" drugs or miraculous results?

Asthma is a sad example of a failure of modern medicine. Drug company cash registers are filling with the money brought in by each new "miracle" treatments for asthma. Yet, each year more people, mostly children, are diagnosed with the disease - and more die.

Overall asthma incidence is rising to epidemic proportions. Asthma death rates are tripping alarms in the medical community.

The asthma problem is especially disturbing because it is a preventable disease. Alternative, safe, natural treatments are available.

While more research into asthma is needed, we already know enough to help thousands of sufferers.

Chapter 35

Digestive Wisdoms –
Fixing your belly ache

Digestion simply means breaking down big things, let's say a rutabaga, into little things, the rutabaga's component parts. Rutabagas, as well as all other foods, are composed of macronutrients, including protein, carbohydrates, and fat, and micronutrients – vitamins, minerals, and everything else. The role of digestion is to break down foods into tiny pieces so they can be absorbed and transferred into the blood for delivery to cells.

Food in your digestive tract is of no true benefit until it enters your cells. All the action takes place in cells. Food must be broken down so it can pass into the blood system which is the highway that takes nutrients to cells. The bottom line is the best food in the world does you no good if it's not digested and delivered.

The most common digestive problems, even life-threatening ones such as peptic ulcers and intestinal cancers, are known to be associated with poor eating habits.

Ulcers

For years, the medical establishment claimed that ulcers were caused by stress. Their theory was that stress stimulated the excretion of excess gastric acid. You might have heard, "Acid eats holes in the stomach." The solution for this simplistic explanation was to prescribe antacids. Stronger and stronger antacids have been developed by the drug companies and are widely advertised. Millions of them are sold every year, even to children. Antacids of various kinds are the largest selling over-the-counter and prescription drugs. "Acid stomach" is so common that drugstores devote entire sections to over-the-counter medicines.

However, did you know that studies do not show that people with ulcers make more acid than anyone else? Why would acid "eat holes" in some peoples' stomachs and not others? After all, we all have the very same acid in our stomach – it's necessary for digestion. Seems to me there's a hole in the theory of acid eating holes.

A newer theory of ulcers is that they are caused by a bacterium in the stomach. Taking antibiotics is now the cure many doctors prescribe, along with an antacid. But, what about the people who have the bacteria, called Helicobacter pylori, but not the ulcer? And what about the people who have ulcers, but not the bacteria? These states are quite common. Certainly no one suffers from ulcers because they're deficient in a drug that interferes with the natural production of stomach acid.

While these and other theories are formulated and turned into a huge profit-stream, naturopathic physicians have been successfully treating ulcers with diet and life-style suggestions.

Healing with Wisdoms

For those willing to look beyond what the drug companies are saying, there is scientific research that supports age-old healing processes.

- Slow down, you eat too fast.

A common lifestyle problem that contributes to ulcers is stress-eating. Ripping into foods and gulping them down denies the natural process of chewing and mixing foods with the alkaline (non-acid) enzymes in the mouth. Research shows that slowing down the eating process, using teeth to break the food into smaller pieces and allowing enough time for salivary enzymes to start the digestive process reduces the incidence of ulcers.

- Fiber vs. Acid.

  Studies have shown that adding fiber to the diet can reduce the incidence of ulcers by fifty percent! Note that fiber is cheap and is not owned by any pharmaceutical company. It is plentiful in the Nutrition 1-2-3 program.

- Feed the gut.

  It's also important to supply the digestive system with the nutrients it needs for growth and repair. The cells lining the stomach, mouth, esophagus and intestines, are subjected to a lot of wear and tear. They need to be replaced daily. Because of this high turnover rate, these new cells require high amounts of nutrients. If the new cells are not strong, they don't stand up well to the acid our stomachs secrete for breaking foods into smaller pieces. By supplying the amino acid glutamine, zinc, vitamins A and E, and flavonoids, the new cells are stronger and more able to resist the acid. The Three Wisdoms program provides plenty of these nutrients and fiber.

Gallstones

Are you now or have you ever been a gallstone producer? If the answer is yes, then you were probably not Regularly eating a Variety of Whole foods.

Gallstone removal is one of the most common

surgeries performed - over 300,000 each year - yet it is completely unnecessary. Hundreds of thousands of people suffer excruciating pain, loss of work and the risk of the knife because the medical-industrial-complex is more concerned about perfecting new surgical techniques than prevention of disease. A gallbladder full of stones is routinely plucked from the body without regard for the fact that it is a functioning organ.

Do you need your gallbladder?

Let's step back for a minute. What is this organ, the gallbladder, which is so quickly and without concern, removed from the body?

The gallbladder, located on the upper right side of your abdomen and suspended from the liver, is a sack-like organ for accumulating and discharging bile.

Bile is the result of an efficient system in which the liver filters the blood, removes worn-out cells, chemicals and toxins, mixes them in a liquid solution and secretes them into the gallbladder. The gallbladder holds this solution until you eat a meal containing fat. Fat stimulates the discharge of bile into the small intestine where it aids in the breakdown of fats. So, the gallbladder aids in detoxification and digestion which is pretty amazing for an "unnecessary" organ.

This is not, however, the whole picture. The gallbladder then performs an even more amazing trick. It reabsorbs ninety-eight percent of the bile and recycles it back to the liver where it can be reused. The unwanted portion of the bile, including many toxic substances, is eliminated with the feces – with the aid of fiber!

The coordinated effort of the liver, gallbladder and intestines is responsible for the elimination of many toxic elements such as fat-soluble hormones, drugs and pesticides. Its fat-digesting function is necessary for the utilization of the fat-based vitamins - A, E and D.

This is a small example of the efficiency of the human

body. Several systems - blood, liver, gallbladder, nervous system, immune system, hormones and intestines – interact together to rid the body of waste, flush out poisons, break down fats and recycle what this system wants to reuse. It's one of the simpler systems of the body, and not nearly as complex as sight, for instance, yet is still a miracle.

The medical-industrial complex, by and large, ignores the miraculous function of the gallbladder. They hold no reverence for the millions of years of evolution that culminated in this system. They ignore their own scientific literature that clearly details the importance of normal bile function and how gallstones can be prevented. They downplay the destructive nature of removing the gallbladder by making the surgery into an almost painless outpatient procedure.

The gallbladder speaks

When your gallbladder hurts, it's trying to tell you that something is out of balance. You can choose to listen or to ignore it. As the gallbladder's voice becomes stronger it might bend you over in pain. Instead of listening and correcting the underlying causes, the business of medicine would have you shut your gallbladder up for good by removing it. Now you don't hear the warning, but the conditions that caused the stones to form in the first place still exist.

Removing the gallbladder doesn't make this system work any better, it only eliminates the source of pain. This is analogous to disconnecting a fire alarm because it keeps going off every time there's a fire.

Naturopaths and other doctors who respect the body's evolutionary wisdom have been preventing and curing gallstones for hundreds of years.

It doesn't take a genius to understand the importance of the liver-bile system. In my experience, most patients who understand will choose to save their gallbladder.

Why do some people form stones?

In addition to what I said above about bile's function, it also regulates the elimination of minerals from the body, mostly calcium. Stones are formed when minerals or cholesterol or both precipitate out of the bile solution. This precipitation accumulates as gravel or stones.

It's elementary to predict why this usually thin, soupy bile solution could change to an unhealthy, thick consistency. Too much cholesterol, too much calcium, or not enough water make for a thicker soup and lead to the cholesterol or calcium accumulating into stones. Another element that causes trouble is inflammation. When the gallbladder is inflamed, bile thickens and stones are more likely to form.

We know from population studies that the factors that increase gallstones include obesity, food allergies, high caloric intake, low fiber intake, intestinal problems, increased estrogen (from hormonal imbalance, hormone replacement therapy, or birth control pills) and drugs such as certain cholesterol-lowering agents. Aggravating factors can be fasting, a high fat intake and coffee.

What you can do about your stones

Because populations who eat traditional high fiber, high nutrient diets do not develop gallstones, many studies have been done to find out why. It is clear that the refined carbohydrate and sugar rich diet of Western countries is strongly associated with stone formation.

Whole foods supply lecithin, fiber, omega-3 oils and natural plant components called terpenes that prevent and even reverse the formation of gallstones. Good old water helps thin the bile soup. Eating Regular meals reduces bile stagnation. Antioxidant-rich Whole foods reduce inflammation.

If you have gallstones, you have a chance of

eliminating them through diet. If you've had your gallbladder removed, changing your diet will do what the surgery failed to do and eliminate the conditions which caused the gallstones in the first place.

Chapter 36

Food Sensitivity Wisdoms –

When Good Food Turns Against You

Food, even real food, and even organic food, may be detrimental to your health. What a thing to say after all the nice things I've said about organic food! Sorry, but life, especially life in the 21st century, is complicated.

Foods can trigger unpleasant chemical reactions. Sometimes these are out-and-out allergies, and sometimes they're not a true allergy but what are referred to as sensitivity. Allergies and sensitivities can be detrimental to your health.

Allergies

True allergies are the result of an antigen-antibody reaction. An example is hay fever which is the outcome of an antigen, pollen, triggering an antibody. An antibody is an antigen-fighting protein that resides on your mucous membranes. The antibody attaches to the pollen antigen because it sees it as being different. Its strategy is to protect you from a strange protein. The antibody is like a good policeman, ever vigilant to head-off injury by stopping bad proteins.

Why does the antibody identify pollen as bad? Because your immune system has evolved to identify any protein that isn't you as a threat. To your immune system, your internal police squad, only you are good and all else is bad. If one of your antibodies catches a foreign protein, it labels it as an antigen and arrests it by holding on tight and releasing chemicals that start an inflammatory reaction. The inflammatory reaction is the swelling, redness and pain you feel when your body is protecting itself from the pollen that landed in your nose. It is also the reaction you would have to a sliver of wood stuck in your finger or if you were given a blood transfusion with blood that didn't match the proteins in your blood.

Inflammation is a natural response to rid the body of a foreign substance. Just enough inflammation results in a sneeze or two. When that inflammation goes too far resulting in a red, swollen lining of the nose with copious discharge and excessive sneezing, the normal inflammation has crossed the line into an allergic reaction. An allergy is, in a sense, the immune system being overly-reactive to the environment. The officer has become too protective.

While pollens are the most obvious example, allergies can also be triggered by foods. Peanuts, for some people, may set off an extreme allergic reaction that is so strong the body goes into shock.

Sensitivities vs. Allergies

Sensitivities are reactions by the body that do not follow the typical antigen/antibody reaction. There is no general agreement on what causes them as there are probably multiple reasons.

In some cases they may be caused by the liver's inability to detoxify a substance. At other times a problem with digestion may allow a larger-than-normal piece of food to cross the intestinal mucosa and travel into the blood. This has been documented by electron micrographs and is known as leaky-gut syndrome. The intestinal flora, or good gut bacteria, also has an influence on how the body reacts to foods, especially sugars.

For these reasons, and probably others, the body becomes sensitive to a food or chemical and reacts with inflammation at each exposure.

It is important to be aware that allergies and sensitivities can trigger anything from a mild to a severe reaction and you can be allergic to more than one thing. The person who is extremely allergic to peanuts may only be mildly allergic to mold, or vice versa. Along with the sensitivity to more than one thing is the potential for an accumulated effect. This is the person who is a little sensitive to wheat and dairy when eaten individually, but when the two are eaten together, he or she suffers an asthma attack.

More than a sniffle –
The many faces of food sensitivities

One of the difficulties with diagnosing food sensitivities and allergies is that they can produce a bewildering array of symptoms.

Research has implicated food sensitivities in the following conditions.

1. Irritation of any mucous membrane

Pain, itching or mucous discharge of the eyes, nose, digestive system, and urinary system are reactions to irritation of mucous membranes. This could manifest as hay fever symptoms when nasal mucous membranes are irritated, or a digestive disturbance from irritation of intestinal mucous membranes, or urinary urgency caused by those mucous membranes becoming inflamed. Many symptoms can result from the inflammation of mucous membranes.

For example, food sensitivities could cause anything

from itchy ears to frequent sinus infections. Or, eating an allergic food might trigger a little gas or a debilitating irritable bowel syndrome. A urinary tract irritation might result in bed-wetting in a child or frequent urinary tract infections in an adult. It is usually worth investigating if allergies are the culprit when a person has a recurrent illness involving mucous membranes.

2. Irritation of serous membranes

Serous membranes are the slick surfaces lining joints. Serous membranes and fluids allow joints to function smoothly. Food sensitivities can cause irritation of these surfaces and result in joint pain. Research with arthritis sufferers has shown a link between metabolic products leaking from the gut into the blood and traveling to joints.

It is not unusual, in my experience, to see some cases of "arthritis" go away when food sensitivities are corrected.

3. Skin rashes

Eczema and other skin rashes may be the result of food sensitivity. Improving digestive function with good bacteria has been shown to protect against and cure eczema in some patients, especially children.

4. Mental/Emotional problems

Food sensitivities have been implicated in depression, learning disabilities, attention deficit disorder, agitation and dyslexia. It's wonderful to see a patient's life-long problem with depression or trouble with reading lift when they remove an allergic food. I've heard people say things like, "The words on the page stopped moving when I found out I was allergic," and, "It was like a cloud lifted from my mood."

5. Lack of energy and energy swings

Fatigue and insomnia can also be the result of food

sensitivities. Patients often describe a "brain fog" that comes over them when they eat their allergenic food.

Diagnosing food allergies & sensitivities

If you're suspicious that you may have food allergies here are two strategies for discovering which foods may be your problem.

1. See a naturopathic physician

State of the art blood testing for allergies is being continually developed and perfected. Conventional allergists usually resort to old-fashioned skin-scratch testing. This has been shown to be highly inaccurate, especially for testing food reactions.

2. Self-testing

If professional help isn't available, it is possible to do a self-test. Have you ever noticed a food causing you any of the above symptoms? If so, this can be a good place to start testing.

Or, if you have no idea what food might be bothering you, make a list of the foods you eat every day. Most people chronically eat the food they're sensitive to because it has a drug-like effect and temporarily makes you feel better before you feel worse.

Statistically speaking, the most common food sensitivities are:

- **Dairy**
- **Wheat**
- **Corn**
- **Eggs**
- **Soy**
- **Tomatoes and potatoes**
- **Citrus**
- **Strawberries**

However, any food, spice, or herb can trigger sensitivities. Be suspicious of any food that you eat daily or that you crave.

Elimination Testing

Once you've identified a food or foods you're suspicious of, leave that food totally out of your diet for at least two weeks. It is very important that you don't cheat. Even a small amount - like the cream in your coffee - can trigger a reaction in a dairy-sensitive person. When you're eating even a small amount of a sensitive food daily, the reaction may be too slight, or become lost in a constellation of confusing factors. During your week of abstinence, keep a daily log of how you feel. Make note of changes in any of your symptoms.

If you are testing dairy, do not eat anything made from milk. That means no cheese, yogurt, cottage cheese, ice cream, or butter. You may eat eggs as they are not a dairy food. I suggest everyone test dairy because it is such a common allergen.

If you find you feel better off dairy, then you can challenge individual dairy foods at the end of two weeks by introducing them one at a time and watching for reactions. You may find that you don't tolerate milk, but do fine with cheese or yogurt.

Watch for hidden sources of the food you're testing. Wheat, for instance, is not just in bread, but in pasta, baked goods, cereals, and many processed foods. The same is true of soy, corn, and dairy. These commonly allergenic foods are found in many packaged foods.

During this elimination week, besides noting if your primary condition improves, watch for any changes in how you feel. You may discover something unexpected. For instance, after a dairy elimination, a patient once told me, "My energy improved by 100 percent, but my rash didn't change." He didn't realize his energy was low until he felt better. It turned out his rash was because of a corn allergy.

Remember, you may be sensitive to more than one food. That means you may feel a little better after eliminating one food, but then feel much better after eliminating a second and third food. For instance, you may have a slight allergy to wheat and cheese. They may only give you a noticeable reaction when you eat them together – for example, the day after the cheese and wheat pizza you feel lousy.

Challenge testing

If after your two-week elimination you're unsure if you're sensitive to a food, try eating lots of it. This is called a challenge test.

Let's say you stayed off wheat for two weeks and you think your knee pain may be better. However, you're not sure because you didn't play your usual game of basketball that week. To "challenge" wheat, after fourteen days off spend a day eating lots of it. If your symptoms become worse, this indicates you have a wheat sensitivity. Watch for symptoms up to 48 hours following ingestion because there is often a delay in onset.

Fasting trial

If you have no idea what you're sensitive to or if you appear to have multiple sensitivities, a Fasting Trial may be necessary.

A Fasting Trial involves going on a severely reduced diet in which you eat only medically prepared hypo-allergenic foods for a period of time. This allows your body to clear sensitivity factors from your blood. After the fasting period, foods are introduced one at a time as a test for sensitivity.

This type of testing should only be done under medical supervision as it is difficult to do and may lead to nutritional deficiencies.

Dairy allergy vs. lactose intolerance

Dairy allergy, that is a true allergen-antibody reaction, can be confused with lactose intolerance. Lactose intolerance is the inability to digest lactose, the carbohydrate portion of milk products. People tend to produce less of the lactose-digesting enzyme, lactase, as they grow older. Babies and people of northern-European ancestry tend to produce the most lactase. Lactase deficiency usually only causes digestive distresses such as gas, bloating, and diarrhea rather than non-digestive symptoms.

The answer to lactose intolerance is taking the enzyme lactase, found in health-food and drug stores, when you eat dairy. Anyone who believes they are allergic to dairy should give lactase enzymes a trial by taking one with each dairy-containing meal.

Curing Food Sensitivities

Even though you are sensitive to a food, you may not be that way forever. While there are certain food allergies that are "fixed," or permanent, such as the severe peanut allergy, many sensitivities can be reduced or even eliminated. Seek out your local naturopathic physician for treatments to reduce your sensitivities.

Some individuals find their reactions to food diminishing the longer they avoid them. This is where the concept of Variety in the Three Wisdom program can demonstrate profound value. A person who is eating a variety of foods is less likely to trigger sensitivity reactions. If you're not eating the same foods every day, the body will have time to "clear" itself before you indulge again. Often people with a mild sensitivity to wheat, for instance, can get away with eating it once or twice a week. On the other days they eat a rotating diet of other starches such as sweet potatoes, millet or rice.

The other way the Three Wisdoms can help allergies

is by encouraging the eating of whole foods without pesticides, herbicides and antibiotics. Some individuals are allergic or sensitive to these foreign substances, rather than the food itself.

The Three Wisdoms also help in another way. Remember an allergy is an over-reaction of the immune system. A whole-food diet, by supplying omega-3 oils, antioxidants and other nutrients that balance the immune system, will reduce the possibility of allergies and sensitivities.

Ellen had headaches

My patent Ellen was a puzzle. She'd had headaches almost daily for years. We tried an elimination diet on her but, "Out of the blue my head starts buzzing, after a while it turns into a band of pain. It didn't change with the elimination trial."

About ninety percent of the time the allergy will be to one of the common foods. Occasionally, I see someone like Ellen who doesn't respond. She'd already seen a neurologist, actually several over the years, and her CAT scans were normal. I also was fairly certain they weren't tension headaches because stress didn't trigger them and they weren't better with massage and relaxation.

When the elimination trial doesn't work, I'll often have my patients get blood allergy tests. They are not one-hundred percent accurate, far from it, but they are sometimes quite helpful. However, Ellen was leaving on vacation and so we decided to postpone the test.

Three weeks later, Ellen returned with good news. "I figured it out! I haven't had a headache in two weeks."

"That's great. What was the trigger?"

"Please don't be mad at me, but remember when I first came in you asked me to eliminate anything artificial from my diet?"

"Yes." I already knew what was coming next. "And, of course I won't be mad at you."

"Well, I just couldn't bear to give up diet soda, I love it. But it was impossible to find in France. So I didn't have any for two weeks and I didn't have any headaches, but I didn't put it together. The day I got home I drank one and as soon as it was in my mouth I felt the buzzing start."

Ellen was definitely sensitive to artificial sweeteners and this is common enough that I ask anyone consuming them, especially when the symptom is a headache, to stop.

Chapter 37

Medical Wisdoms –

Nutrition vs. Drugs

You claim that the Three Wisdom program is good for almost every illness. If disease was this easy to treat, wouldn't my MD teach me about nutrition?

Medicine is a huge field involving years of study. A young man or woman in their early 20's without much experience in the world graduates from college and goes directly to medical school into a residency program. This consists of seven to nine years of learning about drugs and surgery.

Rarely will a student MD have even a brief course in nutrition. If they do, it is influenced by the dairy industry or a multinational corporation that's involved in packaged foods and agribusiness. The results of this kind of education will fulfill the old adage, "To a man with a hammer, everything looks like a nail." You can't expect your MD to function outside the paradigm she or he knows best – drugs and surgery.

The medical-industrial complex and your health

It was President Eisenhower who coined the term "military-industrial complex" to describe the economically-friendly relations and revolving-door jobs between big industry and the military. He felt the boardrooms and the Pentagon were too cozy and warned they needed watching.

I think it is only fitting that, in Eisenhower's spirit, we scrutinize the close relationship between medical industries - insurance, pharmaceuticals, technology, bio-technology, research and advertising - and the medical-delivery systems - individual doctors, hospitals, medical schools and medical associations (the AMA, ACS, ADA, NIS, etc.). These groups form an integrated web of personnel, money and ideology. They are the "medical-industrial complex."

So far the public has been largely uninformed about the close ties between business and medicine. Patients see their individual practitioner as an independent thinker, not as someone whose medical school was financed by big business, who receives continuing-education credit for attending pharmaceutical junkets, whose office closet is full of "free" drug samples and who keeps updated on the latest medical "breakthroughs" by salespeople. (Although they prefer to call them detail-men or women.)

Not that your MD is not sincere. As individuals, most doctors are dedicated to their vision of curing disease. But her or his vision has only seen the hammer - drugs and surgery. In an effort to help their patients, most MDs focus on eliminating symptoms, not curing the underlying problem.

It is not your doctor's fault that the web of business ties reaches deep into university and private research projects. "Independent" research institutions like Seattle's world-renown Fred Hutchinson Cancer Research Center have been caught performing dubious medical trials on unsuspecting patients. Researchers have been charged with promoting clinical trials in which they had a financial interest.

The Fred Hutchinson Center is not alone. Unethical behavior is common, although rarely reaching the mainstream media. Occasionally, someone like Bill Moyers has reported on this travesty for the Public Broadcasting System.

Death from the medical system

You may know that the number one killer in the US is heart disease. But do you know what is number three? Why is it such a carefully guarded secret that complications of drugs and medical treatments - known as "iatrogenic" disease - kill 100,000 to 250,000 people per year? (*Journal of the American Medical Association*, July 2000)

The list of deadly consequences may surprise you: 12,000 unnecessary surgeries, 7,000 hospital medication errors, 20,000 other hospital errors, 80,000 infections in hospitals, and 106,000 non-error, negative effects of drugs. In all, 2.2 million Americans have been seriously injured by the medical-industrial complex. Take into account that

> *"Chronic diseases were all but unknown before the industrial revolution and are the ugly stepchildren of environmental pollution, chemical farming, and food processing."*

these statistics may only be the tip of the iceberg because, according to Medwatch, an independent group dedicated to improving medical care, less than one percent of all serious drug reactions are reported to the FDA.

Please don't say that these deaths are the price Americans pay for having the finest healthcare system in the world - because we don't. According to the World Health Organization, the U.S. has the highest rates of neonatal mortality, infant mortality, number of low-birth-weight babies, and years of potential life lost compared to 13 other industrialized countries. The U.S. also rates low in life expectancy. These are not encouraging statistics from a country that spends far more per capita on medical care than any other country.

The ideology of the medical-industrial complex is one disease/one treatment. How neatly this leads to ignoring the body's natural healing processes and instead looks for a cure that can be patented. This way of thinking is so well ingrained that no one, least of all your busy private practitioner (who sells you, on average, eight minutes of his or her time per visit) questions it. During those eight minutes you give the symptoms and a prescription to stop those symptoms is written out.

It is no wonder that the most frightening and deadliest conditions including cancer, diabetes, and cardiovascular disease have multi-billion dollar medical industries associated with them. The irony, sad but true, is that these diseases were all but unknown before the industrial revolution and are the ugly stepchildren of environmental pollution, chemical farming, and food processing. These facts are ignored as big pharma cranks out patent medicines in a vain effort to find a drug cures for what are social problems.

> *"The ideology of the medical-industrial complex is one disease/one treatment. How neatly this leads to ignoring the body's natural healing processes and instead looks for a cure that can be patented."*

Nutrition-1-2-3 and the Three Wisdoms go to the heart of the causes of chronic disease. They're also simple to follow. Yet contained in their simplicity are millions of years of evolutionary biology. This is a fancy way of saying that these concepts encourage you to eat the nutrients your body chemistry evolved eating.

Many people think that because industrial medicine is complicated and expensive, it's right. Sometimes it is, especially when applied to emergency medicine. Heroic medicine can do great things. I'm glad for it if I'm in a car accident. But when dealing with chronic disease, I will trust the wisdom of my body's evolutionary systems over all the chemists at Eli Lilly.

Live a healthy life while living in the real world

You may feel that the Three Wisdoms, while a good idea, are too perfectionist for your tastes and lifestyle. For some people these involve minor changes to an already healthy eating style. For others, the Wisdoms are a radical change from fries, sodas, burgers and a mindset of not really caring.

My role, as a doctor and health coach, is to help you move in as healthy a direction as you are able and willing.

I offer you three rules for healthy eating. I don't expect you to follow them perfectly, but to become your own boss and to find your own center of gravity, rather than being a victim of the mass consumerism that dominates the food and medical industries.

The encouragement I'd like you to hear from me is:

- o Don't give up on yourself.

- o No one expects you to be perfect.

- o Do what you can each day to respect the wisdom of your body.

- o Live in joy.

Section VI

Dinner conversation –
Tall tales and myths

Chapter 38

Myth -

You inherit disease from your parents

Biochemical individuality, environment and your diet

Jo and Mo are lab rats. They have the same mother, father, grandmother, grandfather, sisters, brothers, cousins, uncles and aunts. They were born in the same litter and grew up in the same cage. They've eaten the same rat chow all their lives. These two rats share essentially 100 percent of the same genetic material. Their life experiences, such as they are, have been identical. They've even run the same mazes together.

Yet, while Jo is all white and heavier, Mo has black spots and was the runt of the litter. What's more, Jo is known by the graduate students that take care of the lab as being more aggressive and a "biter," while Mo likes nothing better than being petted and cuddled.

Why are Jo and Mo, whom you might think would be identical in every way, so different? More importantly, why are you so different from your relatives and what are the implications for this in terms of your health and nutrition?

There are two important concepts to understand: nature versus nurture and biochemical individuality.

Nature vs. Nurture

Since the beginnings of human thought there seems to have been someone asking where we came from and how we turned out like we have.

The "nature" view is that who we are is predetermined by some higher being or law. Depending on the mythology of the time, we might be the product of the influences of many gods, or the decree of one god. Today, the scientific view is that we are the product of our genetic material. Thus billions of dollars are being spent to decode our genes so they can be manipulated for our benefit (and someone's profit).

The "nurture" view is that the people and environment around us has shaped us into who we are. An extreme position on this would be that we are all born blank slates, having no innate nature, and our life script is written by the world we live in.

Heated debates have raged for centuries between philosophers and religious thinkers as to whether we are who we are because of nature or nurture.

Modern scientific thought has bridged the gap and has come to realize that who we are is a shared responsibility of our genes and our upbringing. Yes, we were born with a certain color of eyes, a body type, and even a temperament. However, we also had good parents, bad parents, too little to eat or too much. Some things, like eye color, are not influenced by the life we live. Other things, such as temperament, are definitely influenced by our upbringing. Generally, we are the results of a 50/50 shared responsibility of nature and nurture.

It is the same for most health issues. You may have been born with a healthy set of lungs, but smoked all your life. You may have many relatives with cancer, but chose to avoid cancer risks that you have control over including smoking, toxic chemicals, and certain foods.

Severe genetically-determined diseases

There is a continuum as to how much a gene will influence your health. A strong genetic problem before birth can have a devastatingly profound influence. A 100 percent genetically-determined disease would be one in which you didn't survive the developmental process. An example of a less profound, although still severe, genetic disease is Cystic Fibrosis, in which a child is born with severely defective lungs, but able to live if nurtured with the right medicines, therapy and nutrition.

Even sickle-cell anemia, which is a painful and life-threatening disease caused when a gene codes for an abnormal, sickle-shaped form of hemoglobin, can be influenced by lifestyle. It is a recessive trait, meaning it manifests in those who inherit one gene from their

> *"Most disease conditions are much less influenced by nature than they are by nurturing."*

mother and one from their father. Even amongst individuals who have inherited the two sickle cell genes, however, the disease is not the same. Some individuals suffer much more than others and those with higher levels of antioxidants tend to do the best.

Phenylketonuria (PKU) is a genetic disease that can cause severe mental retardation if the child inherits the two genes that program it. All newborn children are tested for it. The child will become mentally challenged if they eat the amino acid phenylalanine. But as long as they avoid it, they will be unaffected and live a normal life. So, even this hard-wired genetic disease is strongly influenced by dietary intervention.

Unlike PKU, sickle cell anemia and cystic fibrosis, most genetic diseases aren't as clearly wired into our cells.

In Type 1, or juvenile, diabetes, it is believed that this severe form of diabetes is not the result of one gene, but of a series of gene variants and also an external environmental trigger, probably a childhood viral infection.

The so-called "genes for breast cancer", BRCA1 and BRCA2, are actually anti-cancer genes. It is only when someone inherits an abnormality in these genes that she more easily develops breast or ovarian cancer. Not every woman who is born with these abnormal genes develops breast cancer, and not everyone who develops breast cancer has these abnormalities.

Most disease conditions are much less influenced by nature than they are by nurturing. It's common for patients to say to me, "My mother and grandmother both had arthritis, so it's just a matter of time for me." Experience and the medical literature show something quite different though. There are a number of lifestyle factors that either promote or protect against arthritis. The patient's digestive health and intake of omega-3 oils are just two of many known influences on the condition of joints.

> *"According to aging researchers longevity is 70 percent environmental and 30 percent genetic."*

Is your lifespan determined by your genes? According to aging researchers (Science Friday, NPR, Aug 31, 2001) longevity is 70 percent environmental and 30 percent genetic.

What about my family history of _____?

Yes, heart disease, high cholesterol, high blood pressure, obesity, diabetes and cancer all have known genetic influences, but they all are more influenced, for most of us, by what we put in our mouths to smoke or to eat.

Most people are more likely to be influenced by what their parents ate than by their parent's DNA because the majority of us continue to eat the same foods we grew up eating.

Yes, some families have a very strong predisposition toward cancer or heart disease, for instance, but their diet can still tip the balance. Their genetic inheritance may tie them to a shorter leash in terms of being more diligent about eating healthfully.

The So-Called Hereditary Disease

Genetics and genetic predisposition are much pressed in the MD community and by medical technology as being the sole or main determinants in most diseases. This is especially true in regards to heart disease and certain cancers. However, any good geneticist (a scientist who studies genes) or epidemiologist (a scientist who studies the incidence of disease in a population over time) will tell you that your genetic code is only half of the equation. Along with your inheritance, there is also the influence of lifestyle, including your diet.

By studying the health history of twins, researchers have estimated that genetics make, at most, a 30 percent contribution to cancer. Seventy percent of the causes are from environment (*New England Journal of Medicine*, 3:48 2000). Environment, including diet, can change how a gene is expressed.

It is unfortunate that so many MDs pass this fatalistic view of heredity on to their patients. "Because of your family history you must take this medication." Too many patients believe in genetic fate and give up on the many nurturing actions they can take to improve their chances of good health.

It's your choice

Whether your grandparents lived to be a hundred, or died suddenly in their 50s, you have a choice of how you want to nurture your genes. You can abuse the hearty genes you inherited from your grandparents by working in an extremely toxic environment or you can support your weak genes with regular exercise, a healthy attitude and foods rich in antioxidants. The Three Wisdoms are a sound foundation for those of you who, no matter what your genetic code says, believe in nurturing genes and influencing inheritance.

Chapter 39

Myth -

Eating healthy requires more time and money

I won't kid you; healthy nutrition takes more thought and planning than eating junk food. The world is full of easy-to-find, useless, and even poisonous, meals. Bad food is waiting for you on almost every city corner, around every bend in the road and in all nations of the world. However, if you have a sound approach and know a few basic rules, you can eat nutritious, health-giving meals with very little extra effort or expense. By removing the time-consuming element of confusion, you can quickly get on with living a healthy, happy life.

Besides, although it appears quick and cheap to run to your local Fat-Food Outlet (sometimes referred to as Fast Food, but they are one of the biggest causes of excess fat and obesity) you may be wise enough to realize that whatever time and money you're saving up front, you're losing in the long run. A steady junk-food diet shaves years off your life and makes you susceptible to a wide range of diseases including obesity, diabetes, heart disease, digestive disorders, and hormonal problems, to name just a few.

The few minutes and the few dollars a person might save eating junk-food are more than offset by the time they will likely waste and the wages they will lose during their recovery from heart surgery. Even one trip to the emergency room with a gallstone attack will negate all the time you "saved" eating burgers and fries. This does not even include the bending-over-double pain of passing a stone or the psychological strain of a heart attack.

Preparing delicious, healthy meals often takes as little as fifteen minutes, or the same amount of time you'd spend waiting for take-out.

I have no doubt that following the Three Wisdoms will help you feel better; maybe five percent better, but perhaps one hundred percent better. The real question here is not time and money, but the value you place on your health.

Chapter 40

Tall Tale -

Digestion requires careful food combining

Some authors argue that there are laws that govern which foods are best eaten together and which foods should be eaten separately. They call this "food combining." Entire books have been written on various theories of how best to combine foods. For instance, some authors claim that fruits should only be eaten alone and proteins and starches should never be eaten together.

I'm not aware of any scientific justification for food combining. Hunter-gathers were certainly not so fastidious. These rules don't fit with the fact that many foods are themselves combinations. Nuts contain protein, starch and fat. Grains and beans are protein and starch.

The food combining system was proposed by a lay writer a number of years ago and has been perpetuated by well-meaning individuals who don't have a strong understanding of nutrition or physiology. Proponents claim that eating according to these rules is easier on the digestion and that improper combinations cause fermentation in the intestines.

I would argue that if an individual has trouble

digesting food, they should have their digestive systems evaluated by a naturopathic doctor. The problem is probably in their digestive juices, not in the food. A healthy person is able to digest foods in various combinations.

Rather than fuss about which foods go together, stick with Regularly eating a Variety of Whole foods.

Chapter 41

Tall Tale -

Milk is the perfect food

Should I drink milk?

The milk question is extremely common. It brings up several issues: whether the fat in milk contributes to heart disease, and concerns over calcium intake, osteoporosis, and allergies. Let's start with the fat.

Milk fat and heart disease

I may be in the minority about this, but my concern is not over the amount of fat in milk but with the quality of that fat. As with many issues in nutrition, I think most MDs and nutritionists have a tendency to look at milk too narrowly. Because typical grocery store milk has saturated fat in it, they rally for exorcising the evil fat. Let's ask, how much fat is there in milk and is it bad for us?

Of all the possible foods that could be tampered with, milk was an interesting choice. On the one hand you have the powerful dairy lobby claiming it is the "perfect food." They even managed to have it prominently included on the Basic Four Food Group and Food Guide Pyramid posters that are distributed to schools and doctors' offices, even though most people in the world don't drink milk as adults.

On the other hand, the "perfect food" is processed to remove fat. Most nutritionists and MDs mistakenly caution against consuming whole-milk products because they think that "high fat" foods are associated with heart disease.

Why steal fat from milk?

Milk is ideally suited to be tampered with. It's difficult to remove fat from the meat of cows, sheep, chicken and pigs when you keep them in pens and cages and refuse to let them exercise and feed them a fattening diet. Removing fat from milk is quite easy. In fact, fat will remove itself from the milk by floating to the top. Fat and water don't mix, and milk is mostly a watery liquid.

Is milk high in fat?

With the rise of heart disease and its presumed association with eating excess fat, the medical industry urges everyone to lower their intake of fats. It has become almost patriotic to consume low-fat foods. Mr. Jones might not be willing to stop eating hamburgers and French fries, but he feels better about his diet if he drinks low-fat milk.

What nobody ever told Mr. Jones is that whole milk contains less than 4% fat per weight. Milk is mostly water. That's only 8 grams of fat in a cup, although the exact amount will vary with breed, season, feed, etc. Compared to almost every other food Mr. Jones is eating, presuming he is eating the typical American diet of refined and processed foods, milk may contain the least amount of fat!

A 4 oz. hamburger paddy, the "quarter pounder", contains 30 grams of fat. And even Mr. Jones' hamburger buns might contain as much as 4 grams of fat – half as much as a cup of whole milk. Even the lowest "light select" hamburger - which Mrs. Jones occasionally sneaks into her husband's diet - has about 25 grams of fat.

The fat content of many processed foods is as high as or higher than milk. Donuts, muffins, cookies and other foods that many people don't think of as containing fat actually contain more fat than milk. Twenty-four potato chips, depending on brand, may contain as much fat as a cup of whole milk. Bet you can't eat just twenty-four.

Whole milk critics argue that milk is high in fat because 48% of its calories are from fat. It is true, the percentage of calories as fat is high. However, the total number of actual grams of fat is low.

My argument is not that milk is low fat, but only that consumers need to look at hard numbers and realize that milk is mostly water, not fat.

Unhealthy marketing

My guess is that low-fat dairy is more of a marketing gimmick than an attempt to improve America's health. The dairy industry has been over-producing milk for years. Millions of gallons of milk are dumped annually. The industry needs ways to make their product more appealing to consumers. Consumers, although not liking the watery-taste of low-fat milk (at least in the early days when people still knew what real milk tasted like), went along with the processed milk because they thought it was good for them.

Is milk fat a problem?

Maybe more important than arguing about how much fat is in milk is to ask if there is any proof that it is harmful. Between 1970 and 1991 the consumption of low fat (or 1 percent) milk increased by 340 percent. Skim or non-fat milk intake doubled. Butter usage dropped by 25 percent while margarine use grew to be twice that of butter. Whole milk drinking fell by 66%. These are significant statistics.

The campaign to lower milk fat intake was a success.

Even kids on the street will tell you low-fat milk is better for you.

But what good did removing the fat do?

The incidences of heart disease, obesity and stroke have all increased since the introduction of low-fat dairy products. Children and adults are fatter now than ever. Obesity is at epidemic levels. Heart disease is the number one killer.

The latest research supports the fact that it is total calories and not fat that is the biggest influence on health.

It's the quality, not the quantity

Instead of placing so much misguided energy into processing milk, the emphasis should be on eating high-quality organic milk.

It's funny how the medical-industrial-complex is not out promoting organic foods, even though the evidence for their superiority is better established than the need for low-fat milk. Organic dairy products, like organic beef, are higher in omega-3 oils. One study found 500 percent more omega-3 oils in organic milk than non-organic. Organic milk has a better ratio of omega-3 fats to omega-6 fats so it reduces the potential for inflammatory diseases in the body. It has more polyunsaturated fatty acids and less cholesterol than milk from prisoner-cows.

As if a better composition of nutrients were not enough, there are also no pesticides, herbicides and hormones. If only the FDA put as much energy into eliminating artificial hormones from milk as they do removing the fat. If only they cared about the quality of the fat rather than the quantity. Ah, if only...

The only benefit of giving hormones to dairy cattle is to the drug manufacturers. These deadly hormones are getting into our systems, into our children and into the environment. The results, in brief, are disruptions of hormone cycles, premature puberty and derangements in wild animal and fish life cycles. Hormone-related cancers are also increased by this unnecessary pumping of hormones into our systems.

Non-organic cheese is even worse than milk because it is higher in fat which is where the toxic elements are stored. Drinking organic milk and eating organic cheese would make a much greater impact on a person's health than just removing milk fat.

Ignoring the real enemies

While the medical industry has been busy attacking whole milk, they have virtually ignored the health problems associated with sugar and refined carbohydrates. There is far more evidence against these processed foods. Sugar and refined starch are the leading causes of obesity, heart disease, diabetes and most of the health problems of our age.

Milk, calcium and bone health

Yes, dairy products contain high amounts of calcium. Yes, calcium helps prevent bone loss or osteoporosis. But, does milk calcium help with osteoporosis?

In most cultures around the world people do not traditionally drink milk and suffer far less osteoporosis than milk-drinking societies.

Dairy milk consumption is high only in Europe and America where osteoporosis is also high. Asian cultures traditionally avoid dairy. And humans are the only species that partake in drinking milk after childhood.

Other factors for bone health

Bones rely on many factors to maintain strength. Calcium is important, but so are protein, phosphorus, magnesium, boron and vitamin D. Besides nutrition, bones need exercise. Bones grow by being stressed. Take a football player and put him in bed for a week and his bone calcium will drop like a rock.

Stress has a negative effect on bone quality. And imbalances of estrogen, testosterone, growth hormone, insulin, and glucagon can negatively influence bone density.

When you look at the whole picture (instead of just dairy), osteoporosis is more likely the result of a multiple of nutritional and life-style factors. Calcium does not stand alone.

Other sources of calcium

Interestingly, the foods other than dairy that are high in calcium are the foods that are most neglected in American diets: fish with bones, green leafy vegetables, turnip greens, kale, broccoli, various beans, seeds, and whole grains. Sound familiar? A can of sardines with bones has more calcium than a cup of milk. So too does a cup of cooked collard greens or three ounces of tofu. These are not trivial amounts. When did a doctor last suggest you eat more greens?

> *"A can of sardines with bones has more calcium than a cup of milk. So too does a cup of cooked collard greens or three ounces of tofu."*

Vitamin D is low in people living in northern climates and even in those living most of their lives indoors in southern climates. Sunshine hitting the skin triggers the manufacture of this important vitamin which in turn increases the utilization of calcium.

Boron, a trace mineral, is receiving more attention for its positive effect on bone formation and preventing calcium loss in postmenopausal women. It is high in... want to guess? Yes, green leafy vegetables, beans and fruit. Ah, the wonders of real food.

Milk intolerance and allergies

Milk is not a food without problems and I rarely recommend my patients start drinking it if they don't already. Some people have very real problems with milk. They may not digest it because of a lactose intolerance or they may have an allergy.

Milk or lactose intolerance

A fairly high proportion of the population can't digest lactose, the sugar in milk. They don't make the enzyme for breaking lactose down. This can cause mild to severe abdominal symptoms such as gas, bloating, diarrhea, constipation and even severe pain. The intestines become inflamed and this interferes with the digestion of other foods.

In the U.S., the rates of the inability to digest milk, called lactose intolerance, are estimated to be 79 percent of Native Americans, 75 percent of African Americans, 51 percent of Hispanics, and 21 percent of Caucasians. In Asia, Africa and Latin America, the rates are between 15 to 100 percent.

Dairy Allergy

Milk allergy is very common. This is different from an inability to digest it. An allergy is a negative reaction to a food. Technically it is an antibody-antigen reaction, like a reaction to pollen or animals. A milk allergy may cause a variety of problems from nasal congestion to indigestion, fatigue, headaches and joint pain.

Other dairy issues

Patients have a lot of questions about dairy. Here are several other concerns that need to be mentioned.

Contamination

Milk is 88 percent water. The water in non-organic milk is contaminated by the dairy industry with artificial growth hormone, antibiotics and pesticides. Milk becomes a means for a cow to rid itself of these insults to your health.

One-half of the antibiotics produced in the U.S. are applied to livestock. Penicillin is commonly used in dairy herds. Spot checks by the USDA have found ten-times the allowable levels in milk. Humans with a penicillin allergy have been known to react to traces of the drug in milk.

Sulfamethazine, an antibiotic that has been banned for use in dairy cattle, has been found in one-quarter of milk samples. It is suspected of causing cancer.

Inadequate Fat for Children

Infants need a tremendous amount of fat for proper growth and development. Fat consumption in infancy is particularly important for healthy development of the brain and nervous system. The brain, for instance, is 70 percent fat. Some researchers feel that the lack of adequate good fats for growing children may be partially responsible for the rise in behavioral and learning problems.

Cow's milk has less fat than human milk. Organic cow's milk has a better ratio of fats than non-organic. Like human milk, it is lower in cholesterol and higher in polyunsaturated fats.

Powdered milk

Powdered milk is even more processed than low-fat milk. The protein and fats are subjected to high heat during the drying process. This heat damages protein and oxidizes fats. Oxidized fats are associated with atherosclerosis.

When you read labels on processed foods you will find that many of them contain powdered milk. This is just another reason to avoid processed foods.

Milk and ulcers

Some people still believe that milk is a good remedy for treating ulcers. But researchers have found the opposite to be true. Milk stimulates the release of stomach acid. If a person has a dairy allergy or is lactose intolerant, milk irritates the digestive system.

The Dairy Dilemma

When asked about drinking milk, this is what I say to my patients:

- Humans have only been eating whole dairy products for about 10,000 years. This is a relatively short time in human evolution. It is believed that hunter-gatherers did not use dairy except in very limited amounts such as reindeer and goat milk.

- If you consume dairy products now and are healthy, then it is probably okay to continue.

- However, be aware that allergies and lactose intolerance are common and sometimes the symptoms are subtle. Symptoms range from vague digestive complaints such as diarrhea and cramping to such non-digestive symptoms like fatigue or learning disabilities.

- A healthy diet, despite what the dairy lobby says, does not require drinking milk. Two of the major professed benefits of milk, vitamins A and D, are not part of milk naturally but are added in artificial form. Calcium is available from other foods and there are other factors that also affect bone health.

- If you are going to consume milk-based foods, you are better off eating whole milk and dairy products just as your ancestors did in whole, fresh, organic form from truly contented animals.

- While many doctors will disagree with me, removing fat from milk is an unwise tampering with nature. There are other reasons to avoid milk products, but the fat content is not one of them. When in doubt, choose whole foods.

- Remember Variety: If you do eat dairy products, rotate them through your diet, just like you do with all foods. Variety helps keep your diet healthy.

Chapter 42

Myth -

Scientists know better than fish

A fishy story

What looks like a fish, swims like a fish and smells like a fish, but is really a bag of toxic chemicals? Farm-raised fish.

After polluting all the oceans, damming access to breeding grounds, destroying reefs and killing off several species of fish, someone came up with the "solution" of raising fish in floating pens and feeding them an unnatural diet. This is supposed to be progress.

Environmental Disaster

Yes, the oceans are polluted, but fish farming concentrates the pollution even more. Think about it - thousands of fish are kept in confinement. Food is tossed in for them to eat. Uneaten food and fish waste sinks below the pen. Fish farms have been referred to as "floating hog farms."

In some cases fish are brought into a region where they don't normally live. Atlantic salmon are raised in the Pacific Ocean. These fish sometimes escape where they compete with native species. No one knows all of the long-term implications of this, but in most cases, moving species means trouble and is often disaster for the ecosystem.

Poison Fish

Many uninformed consumers believe they're making a healthy choice by eating farm-raised fish. Unfortunately the opposite is true.

Numerous studies have shown that higher levels of mercury and other toxic metals are present in farm-raised fish. Likewise, they have higher concentrations of pesticides, herbicides and other man-made chemicals. Remember, they are not being fed an organic diet. Whatever impurities contained in their feed are being concentrated in their fat stores.

Because of their poor living conditions and unnatural diet, farm-raised fish are more prone to disease. For this reason they are given antibiotics, just like non-organic chickens and cows. Eating these fish gives you a dose of antibiotics which suppresses your immune system, and sets the stage for antibiotic-resistant bacteria to infect you. The American Medical Society considers antibiotic-resistant bacteria a major health hazard. These bacteria are responsible for the death of several thousands people per year in the U.S.

One of the key reasons to eat fish, especially salmon, is for the omega-3 oil content. Because farm-raised fish are not eating their native diet, they have much lower levels of these healthy oils. Last of all, because farm-raised salmon look gray and unappetizing, they are fed a red coloring to fool you into buying them. Most states do not require labeling so consumers are uninformed.

The best and the worst of the wild

Wild fish can be contaminated with whatever is in their water. In general it's a good idea to restrict consumption of fish from lakes, inland rivers and coastal waters. This would include bass, marlin, pike, shark, swordfish, tuna, catfish, carp, flounder, mackerel, striped bass and shellfish.

The least contaminated fish are likely to be from cold water mountain streams and oceans and include varieties such as haddock, halibut, cod, grouper, monkfish, ocean perch, pollock, orange roughy, salmon, and snapper.

What you can do

Your best choice is to eat wild fish from the cleanest waters a maximum of three times a week. Also, please let your government agencies know that long-term ecologically sound solutions are needed. Fish farming should not be tolerated. Stop fish from being turned into feedlot animals.

SECTION VII

Apéritifs

Chapter 43

Who loves you?

Supporting the Wisdoms

The Three Wisdoms eating plan will change your health for the better. I have no doubt about that and I'm supported by the historic record and the best nutritional research. However, I never said that implementing the Wisdoms would be without effort. While the concepts are easy – Regularity, Variety, Wholeness – change is always a challenge. The best things in life often require effort. Are you worth it?

The rewards for changing your diet will be great, but you're defying much of modern culture. You may be changing family traditions or questioning your physician's suggestions. You will definitely be bucking the medical-industrial complex, the agricultural industry, and the multi-million dollar food and beverage industry. Some of your friends may even feel threatened by your healthier way of eating.

If the Three Wisdoms program is a radical change from your usual way of eating, I suggest you recruit support.

I hope you believe that feeling mentally and physically better is a goal worth attaining. It is more likely accomplished if you involve other people. Certainly you want to feel better for yourself, but you also want to be a better person, spouse, parent, child and citizen. You are part of a community. That community might be large or small. Your community is the best resource from which to draw support.

Identify your support community

This is a simple and useful exercise. Make a list of the people in your life that are potential supporters of your lifestyle change. It can be done in your head, but writing things down often helps to solidify them. Writing this list may involve some tough decisions. There may be old friends or close relatives that do not qualify as true supporters. They may actually be sabotaging your progress by encouraging un-healthy behavior. You must decide. If in doubt, talk to them. They may be willing to change their behavior.

Unhealthy eating habits are often based on addictions as well as socialization factors. The drinking buddy who likes you intoxicated, but is scarce when you're sober, is not a supporter. Your "sugar high" buddy may feel abandoned if you kick the sugar habit. On the other hand, talking to your drinking or junk-food buddy might help turn both of your lives around. By the way, I'm not saying you'll never drink alcohol or eat sugar again as long as you live. The goal is for you to take control over when and where you take a holiday.

When you stop or cut down on eating junk food you will find some people supportive and others resentful, critical and unhelpful. It's a natural reaction. After all, you are moving forward and leaving them, so to speak, behind. You are also associating or implicating them in "bad" behavior, although this is not your intention. Depending on their personality and level of addiction, they may make fun of you, turn away in anger, or do whatever they can to tempt you back into the fold. On the other hand, they may be eager to help you through a difficult transition and be ready to join you on the road to health, especially after they see how well you're looking. Be proactive. You pick the restaurant.

Don't be afraid to look beyond your closest friends

and relatives. You may encounter someone at work. That guy who always brings his own lunch and has sprouts in his beard is a likely candidate. When I used to work in hospitals, which are notorious for unhealthy food choices, I would often be taken aside and asked questions from co-workers trying to break away from junk food.

Talk to your supporters

Have an honest discussion of what you're planning and why. It will be more meaningful to them if they know the depth of your sincerity and your motivations. If you feel comfortable about it, tell them about your health problems and why you want to change your eating habits.

If there is some specific action you want them to take, be clear about it. "I know you mean well, but please don't offer me your potato chips." "Instead of sitting here and drinking coffee, would you like to go for a walk once a week?" Be specific. Gives them something concrete to respond to.

Sharing the Three Wisdoms

What many people like about the Three Wisdoms is that it's so easy and logical to explain. No elaborate theories, fads or cults, but good science built on a sturdy foundation of historical record.

- Our ancestors Regularly ate a Variety of Whole, organic foods.

- Nutritional research supports the Regular intake of a Variety of Whole foods.

People, in my experience, find that the Three Wisdoms ring true. They may not be able to implement them on their own, but they want to. With your help, maybe they will.

Don't be made to feel like a failure

In terms of health, fitness and feelings of well-being, many people are made to feel like failures.

According to advertising, you are expected to drink Coke, or Pepsi, and eat some form of high-calorie processed food and be excited and happy with all your laughing friends.

On the other hand, you should be jogging 10 miles a day and eating only low-fat, no-cholesterol foods. And, by the way, you weigh too much no matter what your weight is.

Sound familiar?

Advertisers and the press present a no-win situation - for you. But it's a win-win situation for the food and beverage industries that want you confused, frustrated and, most of all, hungry.

Your agenda, not theirs

The food, beverage and advertising mega-businesses have their own agendas. Those agendas are screamed at you a thousand times a day by radio, TV, printed material, billboards and package advertising. If you do not have your own agenda, theirs will literally take over your mind.

So, have an agenda, a personal goal or resolution of your own. There are many ways to arrive at one. There are lots of good workshops, books, and articles to help you. But don't just pick one off the top of your head. Before deciding on a personal agenda, take the time to think, feel, smell and breathe with your potential goals. The best personal goal will be specific, and not vague.

Make a list and check it more than twice

A good way to start on your personal agenda is to make a list of several possible resolution ideas and sit with them, contemplate them, and then decide which one or several makes the most sense. Find the fit that will affect you most deeply.

Look to your core

To make your agenda strong, it must run deep. The list of possible agenda items must be connected with something that is meaningful to you.

"I want to lose weight so I look better," only scratches the surface. Look better for whom? Why does it matter what they think?

My most motivated patients are the ones who want to become healthier because of loved ones – spouse, children or grandchildren.

Simple goes a long way

Your resolution does not have to be difficult or complicated. Often the simplest changes are the most rewarding. I've seen patients choose and follow through with one simple resolution and have it profoundly change their life. Your resolution might be something as straightforward as deciding to eat a protein breakfast. That one seemingly insignificant change could mean you're suddenly providing your body with the energy it needs make you feel alive. Drinking eight glasses of water a day is another good, easy way to start implementing healthy change. Don't underestimate the power of simple, self-directed change.

Examples of the power of simple resolutions

Jimmie, a 45 year old single parent who felt she had no time for anything, resolved to drink two quarts of water per day (not just "Drink more water" but a specific amount). As a result she found she had more energy, lost 12 pounds and increased her self-esteem.

I've had many patients follow through with a resolution to take a high-quality nutritional supplement twice daily. Most of them feel better after one month. I remember Gary, a business executive, who found he was more calm, less irritable and soon won a promotion at work.

Kim, a teenager, changed her life by resolving to eat four servings of vegetables daily. Implementing this one simple plan decreased her intake of junk food which resulted in the clearing of severe acne. Note her plan was positive and specific: eat four servings of vegetables a day, and not negative and vague: cut down on sweets. (Note: A serving is one-half cup.)

Ten tips for keeping resolutions

1. Take the time to carefully consider, research, and contemplate your potential resolution.
2. Set goals that are your personal goals not someone else's.
3. Set realistic goals that you have a good chance of accomplishing.
4. Have in mind simple, concrete steps for accomplishing your goals.
5. Find support from books, friends, family, your church, and so forth.
6. Vary your routine to avoid boredom.
7. Reward your progress. Positive reinforcement works the best. The rewards should be consistent with your goal (i.e. don't use chocolate cake as a reward for eating more vegetables - that's sabotage). Make your reward something concrete and lasting such as a special book or article of clothing.
8. Learn from your mistakes as well as your successes. Don't look at poor food choices as defeats, but as opportunities to continue improving.
9. Revise your plan if necessary, but do it with a careful consideration for your goal.
10. Try again. Plan B is often more successful than plan A.

Chapter 44

The Power of Positive Eating –

Sitting, chewing, laughing and lingering over meals

The French tradition

We call it the French cholesterol experiment. It was a very non-scientific study involving one person, a friend of mine. There was no control group. The "experiment" came about somewhat by chance.

My friend, Lisa, was 38 years old. She lived a good, but stressful life in Seattle. She was a petite woman who exercised regularly, even ran a marathon and took part in the annual Seattle to Portland bike race several years in a row. The problem was that her cholesterol was always high. It was three hundred and seventy-five on several readings even with all the exercise and a good diet.

She wasn't a junk-food kind of gal. She and her husband, a physician, loved to cook, and were very aware of good nutritional habits.

Then Lisa's life changed dramatically. Her husband took a job in Paris. About a year after settling into a left-bank apartment, I visited them. Coincidentally, Lisa had her blood drawn for a cholesterol check the day I arrived. She was sure her cholesterol would be worse than ever.

The next day we sat in their kitchen discussing the results. As I recall, we'd just finished eating two elegant mini-pizzas with cheese, pesto and delicate vegetables. Susan's cholesterol had dropped seventy points to one hundred and ninety.

We wanted to figure this out. Lisa was exercising less. She never ran any more, although their apartment was a fourth-floor walk-up (Or was it fifth? At times it seemed like ten floors up). She was eating rich French cooking. Although she wasn't under the stress of school, she felt stressed by the move, her lack of a job, learning French and numerous other issues. I remember her telling me, "I know it seems crazy, but I feel more stressed here, because of the uncertainty."

We sipped a fine French wine and discussed the cholesterol problem further. Was the lab wrong? No, a later test confirmed the results. Was there something in the water? This was unlikely. What about the amount of wine? No. She had been a light wine drinker in Seattle as well.

We nibbled on an éclair from the neighborhood bakery, sipped an after-dinner apéritif and focused our minds more on this cholesterol dilemma. (Retrospective analysis is well known to be fraught with difficulties.) As the evening floated along we also spoke of the recent election, the popular French sport of labor strikes, old friends and difficult Internet connections. However, the conversation kept coming back to Lisa's test results.

My theory was that her cholesterol was lower because she was now eating extra-virgin olive oil. Traditionally the French are known for being very particular about their olive oil. Only the first pressing is used. No chemicals are added to aid the extraction. My hypothesis that the high-quality extra-virgin olive oil was the key factor agrees with the research showing that cholesterol levels are lower in countries that use olive oil.

Lisa's husband, Brad, had another idea. "Maybe it's because of what we're doing right now. Since coming here we've adopted the French style of eating. We eat several courses, fairly slowly, over several hours, while we talk and laugh."

Brad was on to something. It made perfect sense from a metabolic point of view. When you eat quickly, which Americans are famous for, your food is going to flood into the bloodstream faster. Once in the blood, the calories are going to rush out to cells. The cells are overcome with too many calories swarming in too fast. This flood of calories will be shunted into cholesterol for storage until something can be done with them.

In Lisa's case she'd often had to eat on the run in Seattle-even in the car on the way to class. You can argue whether she had more or less stress in Paris or Seattle, but one thing for sure was that the stress in Seattle involved more time constraints and deadlines. To help meet these time problems, she ate hurriedly.

"Lisa's situation is an example of a good reason to go to a doctor who will look at your total health from a wholistic perspective. A doctor who is narrowly focused on cholesterol readings will simply say to limit fat intake or take a pill that reduces cholesterol. It's much more useful to look at all the things that can raise cholesterol."

Another part of the cholesterol dilemma might be explained by something I learned later. Among cholesterol's many functions in the body, (It is, after all, a vital part of the life process.) it acts as an antioxidant. It could be that the kind of stress Lisa was subjected to in Seattle caused more oxidative stress to her body. The higher cholesterol might have been a natural reaction, a way of reducing the oxidative damage. In this scenario, the high cholesterol was actually a good thing. Her body was raising her cholesterol to help deal with the higher level of stress that caused more oxidation.

So, was Lisa's cholesterol down because of her exclusive use of extra-virgin olive oil, slower food consumption, less oxidation, or some other factor? Obviously we don't know for sure. She wasn't about to run the experiment again and change to using corn oil and eating faster. Her lab results and the conclusion of a number of experimental studies support the value of doing all of these things.

Lisa's situation is an example of a good reason to go to a doctor who will look at your total health from a wholistic perspective. A doctor who is narrowly focused on cholesterol readings will simply say to limit fat intake or take a pill that reduces cholesterol. It's much more useful to look at all the things that can raise cholesterol. Besides fat intake there are other factors including excessive carbohydrate intake, poor liver function, too much stress, not enough exercise, and eating too fast. Your cholesterol reading is a symptom that needs to be addressed at its cause. Think of high cholesterol as the fire alarm. If it keeps ringing the solution is not to disconnect it but to find out where the fire is.

Fast food:
A collision course with your health

Super-Size Me is a documentary film made in 2003 about a man who spends one month of his life eating three meals a day at McDonalds. Whenever asked, he agrees to the super-size option. At the end of one month he gained almost 30 pounds and his doctor told him he was in he early stages of kidney failure. He also felt sluggish and his skin looked terrible.

What looks like food, smells like food, and tastes like food, but is really poison? Most fast foods.

In addition, there's the issue of frying. Don't let yourself be fooled into thinking that because your favorite French fries are cooked in vegetable oil that they're good for you. The high heat and instability of vegetable oils actually make them worse for you than foods fried in lard, which is more heat stable. (See Chapter 9, Fats 101.)

Then there's the problem of waste. Whole forests are consumed in making the packaging for fast-food restaurants and processed foods. Further waste and pollution is created when you drive to the place and wait in line with your car engine idling.

Eric Sclosser's book, **Fast Food Nation**, goes into gory details about the societal effects of this sort of eating.

Last, but not least, fast food breaks two of the Three Wisdoms. It lacks Variety, relying on wheat and potatoes as starch sources with soy meal mixed into the buns and burgers to make them less expensive. It also clobbers the Wholeness rule because junk "food" is not whole, fresh or organic.

Fast food, in the long run, is even a waste of your time. You can cook a nutritious meal in the time you spend driving to the restaurant and waiting in line. For each minute you might save, you lose years of life and risk spending future hours in doctors' offices and emergency rooms being treated for high blood pressure, food poisoning, gallstones, heart disease and cancer.

Fast food is very expensive when you factor in all the doctors appointments, medicines, surgeries and missed work it will cause in the future.

Fast-food costs you time, money and health. What about truth in advertising? Let's call them "fat-food joints" or "slow-death drive-ins". The truth is they should be avoided.

Chapter 45

Supplements 101 –

Diet is no longer enough

Doesn't food give me all the nutrition I need?

Food is undoubtedly the best way to get the nutrition your body needs. In food, vitamins, minerals and other nutrients are presented to your digestive system and cells in the same way they have been for thousands of years. Your body evolved to extract nutrients from food.

If you closely follow the Three Wisdoms I've presented in this book - Regularity, Variety, Wholeness - then you're probably obtaining sufficient nutrients to maintain yourself if, and this is a strong *if,* you're healthy in all other ways including digestion; and, *if* you don't take any prescription or over-the-counter medications; and *if* you don't now live or ever lived in a toxic environment. All these situations increase your need for nutrients.

The truth is that few people follow the Three Wisdoms completely. They may follow them 50, 70 or 90 percent of the time, but life is full of nutritional landmines and we all occasionally trip one. This is normal and not a cause to give up. These lapses are, however, good reason to supplement your diet.

The question to ask yourself is; of the 1500 to 2000 meals and snacks I eat in a year, what percentage follows the Three Wisdoms?

Subtract points every time you eat sugar, fried foods, or refined flour products such as pastries. Also subtract when you drink coffee or alcohol or are exposed to cigarette smoke. Do you live in a polluted city or work in a place that exposes you to industrial chemicals? Subtract more points. Do you take aspirin or any other medication?

> *"Our ancestors ate food that was more nutrient-rich than what we eat today."*

Because few people live in ideal circumstances, I encourage the use of a multivitamin/mineral or other concentrated supplemental food.

Am I asking people to be "too perfect"? I don't think so. First of all, our distant ancestors, the predecessors to our genetic code, never ate junk food. They were 100 percent perfect. Even if they occasionally missed a feeding because of weather or poor hunting, they never ate food that robbed them of nutrients. When they succumbed to malnutrition it was from eating too little, not too many empty calories. They didn't fall victim to heart disease or diabetes, but to infections and accidents.

Also, our ancestors ate food that was more nutrient-rich than what we eat today. Genetic manipulation, such as is done with fruits, vegetables and grains, rarely makes them more nutritious. The modern apple is bigger, more symmetrical, less prone to bruising, and better able to travel long distances, but it has fewer nutrients.

If hunter-gatherers ate more nutritious food 100 percent of the time, then we might close the nutrition gap by taking supplements.

Supplement questions

When considering taking a supplement, ask yourself:

- Do I have any special problems that put me in extra need of nutrients?

- Do I have, for instance, a chronic health problem (diabetes, ulcers, allergies, heart or kidney disease), or a digestive system problem (poor teeth, nausea, lack of appetite or weak digestion)? Remember that the Recommended Daily Intake (RDI), in addition to being a conservative estimate, was developed for healthy people. If you're not healthy, you automatically fall outside the RDI, meaning your requirements are higher.

- What is my toxic exposure? Our ancestors weren't exposed to air pollution, water pollution, and the thousands of chemicals that are now released into the ecosystem. You are exposed to approximately 100,000 chemicals, most of which have never had their health effects tested. The body is able to detoxify and eliminate some of these chemicals, but that process requires energy and nutrients. The liver, for instance, which is responsible for cleansing the blood, uses large amounts of vitamin C to do this work. Oxidative damage to the body is limited by antioxidant vitamins and minerals such as vitamin E, zinc and chromium.

For these reasons - our imperfect diet, the lower quality of our foods, personal health consideration, and the increasing toxic load - I suggest my patients use a high-quality multivitamin/mineral.

Do supplements work?

In numerous studies, a variety of health conditions have

been shown to benefit from the use of a multivitamin/mineral.

For instance, a report in *Psychopharmacology* (2000;150:220-225) is typical. In this case one group took a multivitamin mineral for 28 days. The comparison group took a placebo. By the way, the supplement was by no measure "high potency". It was not even complete. It lacked vitamins E and A, chromium and selenium. The participants were healthy people. However, even with these limitations, at the end of the 28 days the supplemented group rated themselves less tired and better able to concentrate. This was one of the first studies showing the benefits of supplements on healthy individuals eating a "normal" American diet.

Multiple Choice

Once you've decided to take a supplement, you have some tough decisions to make. There are literally thousands of brands on the market. More are coming out all the time. It's not easy to find a good quality supplement that's right for you. Here are some guidelines:

Narrow the choices

First of all, remember you're not trying to treat yourself for a medical condition. That's best left to your wholistically-oriented physician. Your goal is to find a nutritional supplement that acts like an insurance policy. It needs to fill in the gaps and lapses in your diet and re-supply you with the detoxifying nutrients that are being used up by living in our toxic world.

I use the term 'nutritional supplements' because I don't want to restrict your thinking to only vitamins. There are many other food factors such as minerals, oils, fibers, enzymes, carotenes, etc. which are also important for your health.

I recommend my patients take a nutritional supplement that covers all of the basics. Unless you have special needs, a good multiple vitamin/mineral will cover the major bases. It's not necessary to buy separate vitamins and minerals that you have to count out each day. Who has the time? One bottle is usually enough for most people. You will, however, need to take more than one per day. All the nutrients you need cannot be compressed into one pill without making that pill too big or difficult to digest.

Are the RDIs enough?

RDI stands for Recommended Daily Intake. They are recommendations of vitamins and minerals for healthy Americans. They were established assuming that most people have the same requirements for nutrients. However, when individual nutrients such as amino acids, B-vitamins and calcium are studied, people show a 2.1 to 7.0 fold difference in what they need. Studies show an average difference in nutrient requirements for individuals is a 4-fold variation. This is twice what the Food and Nutrition Board assumes. There may be nutrients with an even wider range.

Keep in mind that the RDAs were calculated for healthy individuals. There is a great deal of debate over who is healthy. Even using standard medical criteria, ruling out the 30 percent of the population that has a chronic disease such as arthritis or asthma and the 40 percent of that are overweight, there aren't too many "healthy" individuals left standing.

Other weaknesses of the RDA are that they do not cover job or environmental pollution exposure, genetic metabolic defects, malapsorption, smoking, alcohol consumption, or the negative effects of prescription and nonprescription medications.

The RDAs may apply very well to a very small percentage of the population, but it is a widespread misunderstanding that RDAs are adequate for everyone's needs.

Over and above the RDAs obvious shortcoming in

meeting the needs of the majority of the population, they do not address optimal levels for maximizing health, productivity and longevity. Yes, some people only want to "get by," but if you're reading this book you probably want to improve your health as much as possible. The right supplement can help you live a life of vitality.

A supplement that supplies more than the RDAs is an excellent choice.

Quality over quantity

With all the thousands of supplements to choose from, finding good quality is the most difficult task. When researchers go into stores and take supplements off the shelves and back to their labs they invariably find that most do not meet label claims. Some even contain toxic substances. One study found that one-third of 260 imported Asian herbal products contained lead, arsenic, mercury or drugs not listed on the label.

Unfortunately, there is no quality control exercised over supplement manufacturers. (The control over plant and animals used for human consumption is also low, but that's another topic.) As you might suspect, profits are often more important than quality for some companies.

What does poor quality mean for the consumer? At the very least it may mean that the supplement doesn't work. What is worse, however, is that they may be harmful. Time and again I see the results of patients taking inferior supplements. It's not unusual for someone to be taking the "right" supplement for their condition, but not getting better. The reason is often because they've opted for the least expensive and poorest quality product.

Doing your own quality control

It's difficult for the average consumer to make informed decisions about the quality of a supplement they're considering, but it's not impossible.

If the product you're considering has any binders, fillers, dyes or artificial ingredients, eliminate it. You're exposed to enough chemical poison already.

Supplement questions to ask:

- Do you have independent assays performed on your products?
- Will you send me a copy of the assay? (An assay is simply a scientific test to verify the ingredients in a product.) Any reputable company will be doing assays regularly and will be happy to supply you with copies.
- The best companies will adhere to Good Manufacturing Practices (GMP). This is currently a voluntary program. This certification means the supplement company is volunteering to adhere to higher standards. ISO-9000 is another certification demonstrating a higher standard.
- Or, you can go to a naturopathic physician who can help you find the exact supplement you need and the quality you deserve.

One thing that helps narrow your search is the internet. Most companies now have web-sites and e-mail. Don't be taken in by the eye-popping graphics and exclamations of "highest quality, all natural," etc. A good web-site allows you to ask questions and even to see the results of independent testing.

I'm not saying that companies that don't have independent assays are not supplying good products or trying to cheat anyone. I'm just saying that without the assay they have no way to prove their product is what it says.

Ideally, when a company buys vitamin X from a wholesaler, they will assay it to make sure they received what they paid for. In the case of herbs, they want to make sure they're not contaminated, moldy or have lost their potency due to age. Then, after all the vitamins, minerals and herbs have been mixed and encapsulated or made into tablets, the best companies will test the product to make sure it has retained all the ingredients in the amounts listed on the label. These tests are expensive to perform and many small companies simply don't have the resources.

Are "name" brands better?

Sorry, but the answer is "No."   When the University of Washington did a survey of vitamin E products available in drug stores, even the big names came out far short of the label claims. The Los Angeles Times recently did a study of St. John's Wort showing similarly dismal results. You recognize a "name" because it's advertised, not because of its quality.

What to avoid

If a supplement contains any dyes, preservatives, fillers or binders, forget about it. Look on the label for silicon dioxide, sodium benzoate, propylene glycol, nitrites, dyes, and anything that doesn't sound like a vitamin or mineral. If they add these things, the manufacturer is not too concerned about quality.

Be cautious about any "new" or "improved" form of a vitamin or mineral which declares "greater absorption" or other such claims. If their product is better, they should be willing to supply scientific studies supporting their claims. Mostly what companies provide are testimonials from individuals. These are one person's opinion and should be considered worthless no matter how famous they are. And speaking of celebrity endorsements, most are paid for, which adds to the price of the supplement.

Beware of allergies

Having bad reactions from your supplement? There may be something in there that disagrees with you. The most common problem is allergies or sensitivities. Your brand of choice should say on the label that it contains none of the most common allergens: corn, soy, wheat, yeast or dairy. This means that the supplement manufacturer has (hopefully) not added them. If you're using a brand that says this, yet you're still having an allergic reaction, then there is either something else you're allergic to in them, or they are not really free of allergens.

When a manufacturer says its product is free of allergens that only means they have not added any. Their supplier, however, may have manufactured the raw materials from wheat, corn, soy, yeast or dairy. Or, the binders and fillers may contain one or more allergenic ingredients. In other words, there is a strong likelihood that a product has corn, soy, wheat, yeast and dairy in it, regardless of what the label says. Use caution if you're an allergic individual. By avoiding fillers, binders, dyes and other non-essential ingredients, you reduce the possibility of being exposed to an allergen.

Are the ingredients natural and whole?

There is a healthy trend in supplements to use food sources for vitamins. The manufacturer may, for instance, use a mixture of dried vegetables to create their product. These are often sold in powder form for mixing with water or juice. These are an excellent way of delivering nutrients to your digestive system. Just make sure the source is organic. I have had many companies claim their mix is organic, but not be able to show supporting documentation. Follow the paper trail.

It is better to buy vitamins in their whole, complex form. Vitamin E, for instance, should be listed as a mixture of natural D-Alpha, Beta, Gamma and Delta vitamin E. Most supplements will only contain the D-Alpha. Likewise, with carotenes you want a natural mixed blend, rather than the product with only beta-carotene. It's analogous to taking only one of the B vitamins, rather than the complete B complex.

Should a supplement contain digestive aids or herbs?

The amount of digestive aids such as hydrochloric acid, pancreatic enzymes and papaya that can be added to a supplement is not usually enough to make any difference. If you have a digestive problem, visit your naturopathic physician, find out what the problem is and take something that will truly help you. I am not aware of any studies showing that adding these to a supplement increases the potency. Added digestive ingredients are probably not worth the extra expense.

Herbs are often added to vitamin pills. The consumer looks at the label and says "Wow. In addition to the vitamins, this has all these herbs added! I'm going to buy this one." The reality is that there's usually not enough of the herb in the product to influence a hamster. In the trade this is called "window dressing". The label looks impressive, but actually little benefit is added. If you feel you need gingko or ginseng or some other herb, consult with someone who understands how these work and how they interact with each other to see if they're right for you. Otherwise, you're just wasting your money.

Digestibility

A supplement won't work if it can't be broken down in your digestive system. Pills in the toilet do you no good. In general, but not always, liquids, powders or capsules are the easiest to assimilate. Some tablet manufacturers do a good job, but most do not. In order to get all the vitamins and minerals they want into a tablet they compress it together so hard that it will pass through you and be in the ocean before dissolving.

A simple test you can do at home is to drop the tablet into a glass of water and wait. According to pharmaceutical standards, tablets should fall apart within a half hour at 98.6 degrees Fahrenheit.

How much should a supplement cost?

There is some relationship between price and quality. My experience has been that the lowest priced drug-store supplements and discount mail-order supplements are not very good quality. This includes wholesale warehouse brands.

To some extent, you get what you pay for. Low-cost brands tend to use more of the cheapest vitamins and minerals and less of the more expensive. They also usually compress the tablets so hard that they won't break down. In addition, they're loaded with dyes, fillers, binders and other things you are better off avoiding.

Often different brands come from the same manufacturer. The only difference is the packaging and price. These manufacturers need to produce a lot of product as quickly and cheaply as possible in order to make a profit.

At the other end of the spectrum, many companies charge way too much for what they're selling. Paying more doesn't necessarily mean you're ingesting better ingredients. Often it's the packaging and promotion you pay for. One very popular and expensive supplement company was recently fined by the FDA for false advertising.

As an example, in my office we sell several brands of multiple vitamins/minerals. Because we have so many patients with unique needs, we like having a variety available to choose from. These brands are available to doctors only. They are in capsules, or easy-dissolving tablets, are organic and meet our strict standards of quality. The prices range from $28 to $45 for a bottle. The bottle will last from 30 to 90 days depending on the patient's health needs. That works out to about $.33 to $2.00 a day.

This gives you an idea of about how much you should be paying for a basic, excellent-quality, no-frills supplement. Less than this and you're probably not getting enough quantity or quality. More than this and you may be paying too much. If you're paying more than this, ask a lot of hard questions of the company. If they sell something that is really better, ask for the studies on humans proving it.

It's up to you to decide if you're worth less than $2.00 per day. Are you worth the price of a cheap cup of coffee? If you think you're only worth a discount brand, then I'd skip it altogether. The likelihood is that you're wasting your money and perhaps doing yourself harm with a cheap brand.

I have never seen a product sold through multi-level marketing that I thought was any better than what you can buy without paying to become a dealer. In my experience the prices are just as high or higher, even with the "discount." The main focus of these plans is to create wealth, not health.

Whole Food Supplements

There is a growing trend toward using "whole food" supplements.

I'm aware of two kinds:

- Dehydrated vegetable and fruit concentrates. Dehydration is a natural process that our ancestors used. They come in capsules or powders and are either from a single source, such as pomegranate, or mixed.

  The powders are mixed with water, juice, or into a smoothie. They can provide the equivalent of several servings of fruits and vegetables. Capsules are convenient, but the dosage is many caps per day.

  The shortcoming of either type is that much of the natural fiber has been removed. On the other hand, they can be high in antioxidants. This should be listed on the label. I often recommend a mixed, organic blend of fruits and vegetables to my patients.

- A number of companies promote "natural, whole-food vitamins and minerals." Some of these are yeast organisms that are grown in a particular way. These are supposedly better utilized by the body, but I have not seen any proof of this. The price is much higher than other vitamins. At this time I'd be cautious about spending money on unproven technology. Save your money for organic foods.

Whichever your choice, be aware of possible allergenic ingredients such as wheat, dairy, corn, yeast and soy. I favor a powdered, organic blend of many fruits and vegetables (Variety) with no sugar, fructose or artificial sweeteners and GMP certification. They're very handy for daily use, for emergency "didn't-shop" days, and traveling.

Supplements and the Three Wisdoms

The healthier you are, the cleaner your environment, and the better you adhere to the Three Wisdoms, the less you will need supplemental nutrition. If you do agree that an extra intake of vitamins and minerals is a good idea, find a quality product that is fresh, organic and whole.

Chapter 46

Sprouts -

Fresh, organic, whole food every day!

Why sprout?

Two words: Variety and nutrition. There are many different kinds of sprouts to add to your meals. Sprouting increases protein and vitamin content of seeds and beans.

What to sprout?

When most people think of sprouting, they only think alfalfa or Chinese bean sprouts. However, virtually any bean or seed can be sprouted. The most common sprouts are alfalfa, barley, chia, most beans, clover, fenugreek, wheat, rice, millet, peas, and radish (for a little spice). Use organic seeds. Never use seeds that were intended for planting or animal consumption as these have been coated with fungicides.

How to sprout?

Equipment

- Wide-mouth canning jar.
- Ring lid without the center or a rubber band.
- Cheesecloth.
- Home sprouters are also available commercially.

Method

1. Place three tablespoons of seeds in the jar or sprouter and soak them overnight in pure water. The room should be around 70 degrees or you can keep the jar near a light bulb or pilot light.
2. Attach the ring and cheesecloth and drain off the water. Rinse again with clean water.
3. Rinse the seeds 2 to 4 times daily. After each rinsing, place the jar upside down so the water will drain off.
4. After several days you will see sprouts growing out of the seeds. As soon as they sprout they are edible, but waiting a few more days enhances the flavor and nutrient content.
5. Beware of seeds clumping together. When they do this they won't drain sufficiently and will spoil. Chia, flax, cress and other mucilaginous seeds are the most difficult. Do not eat any moldy sprouts. Mixing large and small seeds helps increase air circulation and reduces mold.
6. After several days of sprouting, they may be placed in a window where the sunlight will help the green chlorophyll develop.
7. Once mature, sprouts can be retained in the refrigerator for several more days. Avoid letting them get too wet or too dry.

What to do with sprouts

Sprouts can be eaten raw, roasted or cooked into soups and stir-fry. Think of them like you might spinach: a low-calorie vegetable that can be eaten raw or cooked. Talk about fresh and full of flavor and nutrients!
Enjoy.

Chapter 47

Is the media making you sick?

Unless you avoid TV, radio, magazines, the internet and newspapers, you're bombarded with health claims for various products. The grocery store is another place you're hit with promises. From simple statements such as, 'low fat,' to the seductive promise of 'removes wrinkles,' we're all exposed and tempted.

What I think we all want is for the products to be presented in a reasonable, honest way. What we get is some advertising executive's version of the truth. Yes, the sandwich may be "low fat" as compared to the burger, but the fat is still quite high and is hydrogenated. Yes, the wrinkles may seem to disappear, but the real problem is oxidative damage.

There is no crystal ball that separates the truth from lies or even wishful thinking, but there are strategies for getting beyond the hype, fads and false prophets seeking profits.

The Three Wisdoms to the Rescue

One of the great benefits of the Three Wisdoms - Regularity, Variety and Wholeness - is that not only do they apply to your daily eating strategy; they can also be used as benchmarks for evaluating health claims.

When you hear on the news that eating more vegetables protects against cancer, or that beta-carotene causes cancer, the Three Wisdoms give you a solid foundation on which to stand.

"Yes," you can say, "eating lots of vegetables probably does protect me from cancer because it fits with the Three Wisdoms - regularly eat a variety of fresh, whole, unprocessed foods."

Let's look at an example. We'll use a hypothetical headline that, knowing the media, probably has appeared somewhere: Carrots cause cancer.

Could this be true?

First of all, you'll remember that the media usually exaggerates in order to stimulate interest. Secondly, you know they have not reported all the facts, but only what they think is "news worthy" and that is, what sells. If you really want to know what the original report says, you'll need to track it down yourself. However, even without knowing all the facts, you can still make some intelligent assumptions about the research by applying the Three Wisdoms.

Let's say that below the headline "Carrots Cause Cancer" you find the news report actually says that beta-carotene, as found in carrots, increases cancer rates. You could start by asking yourself whether it makes sense that beta-carotene, a necessary nutrient for human health, a nutrient found abundantly in nature, would cause cancer. Maybe this is true, but unlikely, unless given in huge amounts.

Then you could ask: was the weakness with the original experiment or with the reporting? Often it's the press exaggerating. Perhaps the original research found that beta-carotene in doses 1000 times the usual intake caused cancer in mice. Well, yes, we can believe that.

If you're looking for an excuse to stop eating carrots, then you take the report at face value. If you know the Three Wisdoms, you look deeper.

Was something about the experiment not in conformity to the Three Wisdoms? What could make beta-carotene appear to increase the likelihood of cancer?

Applying the Three Wisdoms to media reports

Regularity and Variety: was the beta-carotene given in doses humans usually consume or at much higher levels? Even water can kill you in excessive amounts, especially if consumed in a short period of time.

Wholeness: Was it the natural form of beta-carotene? Or did the researchers use a synthetic form? If synthetic, then the research might turn you off to synthetic beta-carotene, not to carrots.

Wholeness: Was the experiment done with the natural mixture of carotenes, as found in nature, or only the isolated (and thereby not whole) beta-fraction, the type most commonly used in supplements?

By applying the Three Wisdoms to this news report, you're less likely to condemn carrots and beta-carotene as bad and stop eating them, but more likely to check your multivitamin and make sure it contains a natural mix of all of the carotenes.

"The media are more likely to report insignificant or limited research outcomes as a "Major Discovery," "Revolutionary Breakthrough," or "Greatly Promising" because these headlines sell papers and promote the careers of scientists, universities, and corporations."

While most reporters may be trying to do an accurate job of reporting on food and health issues, they, like most consumers, are uneducated about the facts of nutrition. In addition they or their editors or publishers are influenced by the fact that their job depends on the processed-food industry.

They also need to "sell" their article and the way this is often done is through sensational headlines.

So, it's not uncommon for a very small, limited, mouse study which has shown negative results to be blown up into, "Carrots Cause Cancer" or whatever other outrageous claim you've read.

The media are more likely to report insignificant or limited research outcomes as a "Major Discovery," "Revolutionary Breakthrough," or "Greatly Promising" because these headlines sell papers and promote the careers of scientists, universities, and corporations.

In the rush for sensational headlines and selling newspapers or magazines, it is not unusual to read this sort of hype about a new "breakthrough" drug that hasn't even made it out of the lab and into a test animal, much less a credible human study.

This sort of drug promotion through media hype is especially prevalent on the business pages. Scientists are keenly competitive. They promote their own pocketbooks as well as egos by releasing carefully worded press releases boasting the potential and downplaying the side-effects of their laboratory manipulations.

The press are also often lacking in full disclosure. For instance, they might quote a doctor as saying "Naturopathic doctors are quacks" without disclosing that the doctor not only has never met a naturopath or looked at the curriculum of naturopathic colleges, but also works for an organization such as the American Medical Association which has a long history of viewing naturopathy as a rival.

Full disclosure is especially important in this era of corporate mergers. If a television news organization is owned by the same corporation that also owns a food company, you can expect slanted or limited coverage of health issues surrounding the food industry. Don't expect an impartial, in-depth analysis of organic versus corporate food production from any major media outlet in the U.S. They are all part of mega-corporations with their hands in shipping, chemicals, agribusiness, packaging, advertising, and food manufacturing.

Example study: All liquids the same

An editor of a popular health newspaper recently asked me to respond to a bevy of news articles that had appeared claiming that research "proves that drinking any liquid, including sodas and coffee, is handled exactly the same as water."

How does this hold up to the Three Wisdoms? Our ancestors drank only pure, fresh water, or natural, wild teas. Knowing this made me skeptical of these reports, so I looked up the original research.

It turns out that this supposedly definitive experiment comparing water with coffee and soda was a one day study on a small handful of people. The researchers even called it a "pilot study" meaning that the only thing you could conclude is that more research needs to be done to prove anything. This didn't stop the experimenter from bending the media's ear about her (premature) conclusions.

Furthermore, while it was true that hydration, as measured by comparing the participants' weights before and after the one day test, showed no statistical difference, there were differences in other parameters such as sodium and potassium. But these were not reported in any of the mainstream media reports I read.

Why was this little pilot experiment with contradictory results given so much positive press? I can't help but think that maybe the news media was influenced by the propaganda efforts of the study's sponsor: The Coca-Cola Company.

Evaluating the next big diet

What about when a co-worker tells you about the "fabulous"

diet he's on? This person feels great and has lost ten pounds in two weeks. He's eating a no-fat diet (or no protein, or no carbohydrates, or only fat, only protein or only carbohydrate diet, whatever the current best-seller is preaching). Are you tempted to jump on board this fad-diet train? Not if you apply the Three Wisdoms. They make spotting unbalanced diets easy.

You know your friend's diet, even if it is a best-seller, goes against what is known historically and scientifically about good nutrition. Eating only one food or one class of foods does not fulfill the body's requirement for Variety.

If you're brave, you can try to convince your friend of his folly before he finds out the hard way, although some people have to learn through experience.

Books, book tours and book promotions can also be part of the corporate hype. Chain bookstores often have agreements with major publishers to display their books in prominent locations. It's no wonder that certain author's books become best-sellers over and over, regardless of the quality of the writing. Because they have sold well in the past, their publisher knows that advertising and book placement in chain stores will send them to the top again. This is mostly a phenomenon in fiction, but certain non-fiction authors are also highly-promoted by their publisher.

If a book touting the wonders of a drug is published by a publishing house that is owned by the same multi-national corporation that also sells the drug, then you can expect that book to be promoted, a book tour launched, and to hear interviews with that author on your local TV and radio station. Notice how many books are published and promoted on the benefits of Prozac?

Corporate Connection

The food industry spends billions of dollars every year promoting their products. It is an industry with a capital "I" and that stands for them over you. It is not a "We" business.

It is not a farmer bringing produce to market. It is trucks, processing plants, bottling facilities, animal-rendering plants, canning factories, labeling machines, forklifts, warehouses, advertising specialists, distribution networks, wholesalers, and retailers. Your health is up against an army.

Corporations have little interest in bringing anything resembling a natural food to market. There is not enough profit involved in broccoli, potatoes, or apples. What they manufacture are food products - a food with a lot of "value" added. Read, profit.

It's not that corporations are intentionally sabotaging your health, but their business goal is making money, not promoting health. Their bottom line is profit and stock price. Each of the individuals doing the dozens of jobs that transform a whole potato into a box of chips may be upright and loving people. The truck driver, machine operator, food chemist, advertising writer, and corporate CEO may be decent in their personal lives. But their jobs, as have been defined and they have accepted, are to bring a product to market and have it sell. They have no vision of any greater good, no whole-earth perspective of a healthy planet with healthy people. They are willing to box themselves into a world view that is destroying the planet and your health. Don't buy into it.

An important first step in building a healthy diet is to disregard at least 75 percent of what the media says and to do just the opposite of what the food industry wants you to do. This may sound like an exaggeration, but think about it. The food industry (and by this I mean the corporations responsible for chemical farming, processing, packaging, and shipping of foods) are responsible for most of the advertising. You don't see advertising for whole potatoes. Television, print, and radio insult us with sliced, diced, pressed, fried, salted and preservative-laden potatoes.

By not consuming corporate garbage (most of it is not "food," but "anti-food"), you are contributing to the health of yourself and the planet.

Fortify yourself with a solid foundation

You are not alone in feeling at the mercy of all the "experts" who write books, neighbors who preach the merits of a popular diet and news reports of "the facts." Most people do not have the knowledge or the analytical foundations to separate fact from fiction.

Arming yourself with the Three Wisdoms gives you a powerful tool to use against consumerism, fraud and bad science.

Chapter 48

Finding Doctor Right

The medical system in the U.S. is upside down. Too many people go to specialists when they should be seeing a generalist. The ultimate generalist is a naturopathic doctor or a wholistically-oriented MD.

Wholism in health

Ecology is a system in science that takes into account multiple aspects and processes of our environment. It looks at your local lake, for instance, as an interacting system involving rain, plants, animals, drainage, human encroachment, and so forth. This is a wholistic way of looking at the health of your local environment.

The same principles of ecology and wholeness also apply to human health. 'Holistic' health is now used in advertising campaigns for health insurance companies. They know there is enough positive association with the word to lure customers. As with their lack of knowledge of the Spotted Owl, most patients and doctors have little understanding of the specifics of looking at the body as a unified whole. Even the word 'holistic' sounds more like the description of a black hole in the universe rather than a 'whole system.'

A wholistic approach to health means looking at

patients' physical signs of illness, their body chemistries, the environments in which they live, their exercise, family lives, and jobs. Everything in a person's life, from the lead-based paint they chewed on as an infant to the present lack of sleep, influences health. The more of this information that can be examined and integrated, the more likely we are to affect positive health changes.

I believe the best doctors are the ones that are willing and able to integrate all the issues of your health and collaborate with you on a comprehensive plan for maintaining or reestablishing wellness.

Three-step medical care

Naturopathic treatment order can be broken down into three stages:

Stage 1: Prevention

Prevention means staying healthy through diet, exercise, education, sleep, love and all the other lifestyle factors that contribute to health. Not nearly enough time, energy, money or research is directed toward prevention. Prevention could be saving us hours of pain and suffering, early death and even trillions of dollars. It has been estimated that adult-onset diabetes, a preventable disease, will cost the U.S. healthcare system three trillion dollars a year by the year 2020. The demand for new technology has pushed true preventive medicine out and substituted the much more billable 'early detection.'

Stage 2: Restoration

If you become out of balance and begin manifesting signs or symptoms of illness, then use natural therapies to restore your equilibrium.

"Natural" is a much abused word. To me it simply means something that restores a person's own, innate, self-healing processes. If you are not producing enough of a certain hormone, don't take a synthetic hormone; give the gland that produces that hormone the nourishment it needs to produce your own hormones. If you're chronically coming down with colds, sinus infections, bladder infections or some other form of infection, then restore your immune system. Likewise, if your blood pressure or cholesterol is elevated, find out why and do something about the underlying cause. Don't just cover up the symptom. Symptoms are fire alarms, or early warnings. Don't just shut them off. Find and treat their cause.

The same can be said for adult-onset diabetes, arthritis and most other chronic health conditions. Determine the cause and treat them naturally. Nurture yourself back to health and avoid the side effects of drugs.

Stage 3: Intervention

If your health is not responding to natural restorative treatments, then consider drugs or surgery under the guidance of an expert. Drugs and surgery should be the last resort, not the first choice in medical treatment.

The obvious exception to this three-stage model is trauma and emergency medicine. Sometimes, in extreme circumstances, drugs and surgery become the first interventions.

The problem with our current system under the control of the medical-industrial complex is that medicine is practiced upside down, as if every health problem was an emergency requiring extreme intervention. This model has created a very expensive system in which the system itself is a major killer.

Finding the right doctor for you

So, how do you find a doctor who practices medicine in a natural, right-side-up manner?

If you're lucky, your state licenses naturopathic physicians (ND). Check your local phone book or do an internet search for your state naturopathic association. If that process doesn't yield anyone, check with the American Association of Naturopathic Physicians (www.naturopathic.org) and find an ND close to you.

If there are no NDs in your area, then you can sort through the yellow pages for MDs, osteopaths (DOs), chiropractors (DCs) or acupuncturists in your area to find someone who is wholistically oriented and has an education in nutrition. Recommendations from friends also can be helpful.

Don't be afraid to ask for a ten minute in-person or telephone interview with the doctor so you can determine if he or she is right for you. Ask her about her education and experience, especially with treating people with your same health concerns. If she is practicing nutrition-oriented medicine, then ask about her training. Some doctors read a few books or attend a seminar and feel they know enough. Others have extensive post-graduate education. Find out how much time she will spend with you on the first and second office calls. Wholistically-oriented physicians usually allow more time than the standard 8 to 15 minute MD appointment.

One warning: MDs generally have no training or background in wholistic medicine. If they have an interest in nutrition or "alternative" therapies they will take classes and attend seminars. That's a good start, but it doesn't necessarily train them to treat wholistically. They often have a tendency to use vitamins and herbs like they would drugs. Instead of looking for underlying causes of disease, they will attempt to treat the symptoms only. In discussing a doctor's philosophy of disease and treatment you can determine if they're oriented toward restoring health naturally.

Chapter 49

More than a once-over –

The lost art of the thorough health evaluation

Part of the process of setting health goals is to first take a thorough look at your current health. There are many ways to do this. Unfortunately in today's fast-paced world, health evaluations are often limited to a brief physical exam and a laboratory screening of blood and urine.

The following are some suggestions on how to make your assessment more thorough. Feedback from family, friends and Wholistically-oriented health practitioners is also essential.

1. Assessment

a. Medical History

Good doctors have comprehensive health questionnaires that you fill out before an appointment. Or, you can find them in self-health medical books. The process of answering personal questions about your health can be enlightening. If you have symptoms, discuss them with your health provider.

b. Family Medical History

Knowing your family's health history can give you clues on

what to work on with your own health. Remember, most diseases are not caused by genes but are only influenced by them. Your susceptibility to arthritis, for instance, is still dependent on how you eat.

c. Physical Examination
Do this with an examiner who is willing and able to talk to you about her or his findings and is knowledgeable about prevention as well as the treatment of disease. Include your waist to hip ratio (See Section IX for chart). This is an excellent indicator of mortality, diabetes, cancer, hypertension and cardiovascular disease. Your body mass index (BMI) and/or percentage of body fat are also important measurements for predicting your long-term health. (See Section IX for examples.)

d. Laboratory Tests
If you're healthy, at least have a basic screen done. This should include a complete blood count (CBC), chemistries, glucose, lipids (HDL, LDL, Triglycerides) and urinalysis. You may also need some specific tests such as thyroid, homocysteine, liver function, digestive function, etc., depending on your family and personal health history.

e. Diet Analysis
What do you really eat? The best way to be honest with yourself is to do a diet diary. Write down everything you eat for a week. You might even want to write down how you're feeling at different times of the day on the same diary (a diet/symptom diary). The second best method is to fill out a food intake recall. Most of us eat about 1000 meals/year plus snacks. What percentage of your meals is healthy?

f. Specialty Testing
Depending on your health and family history, you may want to have specialized testing such as treadmill, gynecological,

mammogram, colonoscopy, pulmonary function, digestive function, etc. These become more important as you age.

g. Exercise Evaluation
Write down an honest accounting of the times and durations of your exercise. Include "incorporated" exercise such as regular use of the stairs at work, walking to the corner store, etc. Most importantly, are you doing something fun that increases your heart rate to over 100 three times weekly for at least 30 minutes? That's a minimum.

h. Toxic Load Evaluation
Are you exposed to chemicals, heavy metals, molds or other toxins during your job, hobbies, or living situation? Or have you in the past? You can be evaluated with a urine toxic metal test. Liver detoxification tests are also available.

i. Happiness Index
How much are you enjoying what you do in life – your home, job, school, friends, and family?

j. Learning Index
Mental health requires keeping the mind active. What are you learning? What do you want to learn?

k. Take a Look
Stand naked in front of a full-length mirror and write down what you like and dislike. (Close the curtains!)

2. Prioritize
After doing your assessment, make a list of your health priorities. What is your greatest concern, fear, danger?
Discuss your priorities with your health-care provider.

a. List current health problems.
b. List chronic health problems.

c. List family health history.

d. List long-term health goals.

Just how often you have a health evaluation depends on your goals, health history and family history. An evaluation once every year or two is a minimum.

Keep copies of your laboratory and other tests. This is handy in case you switch doctors or your doctor loses your results.

Chapter 50

Who do you trust?

Sorting facts from fads

The quality of the food eaten in the U.S., according to numerous studies, is generally dreadful, especially among the poor and undereducated. People who eat the Standard American Diet - SAD - should be living in dread of all of the deadly and debilitating diseases of our modern age including diabetes, all forms of heart disease, obesity, cancer, arthritis, asthma, irritable bowel diseases, premature mental decline and many neurological and psychological conditions, to name just a few. If you are a SAD eater you should know that you are increasing your risks of poor health and an early death.

Most of the population seems completely ignorant of how their poor food choices are undermining their health. Why do the majority of people eat the deadly SAD? Here are a few of the reasons I've come up with.

Why we don't understand good nutrition

Failure of schools

Schools pay little attention to nutrition. When they do they teach it, it's based on models provided by the food industry.

The food industry, while sometimes paying lip-service to eating real food, wants us to eat more processed foods. Just as illegal drug pushers dilute their product so they can make a higher profit; food manufactures dilute and distort natural foods by processing them into forms with less nutritional value and more toxic elements.

Poor school lunches

School lunch programs do a poor job of demonstrating how healthy and delicious good food can be. The food is so bad that tons of it is thrown away each year by children who are in their peak years for needing calories and nutrients. In recent years many schools have given up on their internal food lunch program and have capitulated to the fast-food industry. They have allowed their lunchrooms to be taken over by corporations whose bottom line is profit. The fast-food industry produces the lowest common denominator of processed, unbalanced and toxic meals. Vending machines for colas and sweets only intensify the assault on our children's health.

Poorly-educated parents

Poorly-educated children often grow up to be poorly-educated parents. Parents are often unaware of the health dangers of a nutrient-deficient diet. They don't recognize that their child's frequent respiratory infections, allergies, asthma and learning problems are influenced by their diet. Instead of putting as much effort into their child's diet as they do their sports activity, they turn to MDs for help. It amazes me to see parents spending hours supporting their child's health by helping them regularly exercise through playing sports, and then drive them to a fat-food franchise to celebrate.

Under-educated medical doctors

Medical doctors, who are almost completely lacking in

nutrition education, pressed for time, and dominated by the drug industry, are less inclined to ask about a patient's diet and more likely to write a prescription for a drug that not only avoids addressing the patient's underlying problem, but further undermines his or her health. It's not their fault. MDs are generally well-meaning people. They just don't know any better. They've been taught drugs and surgery; they see no other answers. Drug salespeople strongly influence doctors' choices of prescriptions. Doctors deny this, but research shows it to be true. The pharmaceutical industry knows how doctors make decisions and spends millions influencing what your doctor writes on the prescription pad.

Misguided medical industry

Medicine is a profit-making industry. Its strength is in treatments including emergency medicine, surgery and drugs such as antibiotics that are necessary when the body needs heroic intervention. The medical industry is so completely wedded to heroic treatments that they spend few resources on prevention, in general, and nutrition in particular.

Most people, however, are not suffering from diseases that are best treated by drugs or surgery. They have chronic degenerative diseases like diabetes, Alzheimer's, obesity, cancer, arthritis, digestive problems, heart and vascular diseases that are far better treated by nutrition and lifestyle changes. Heroic intervention is not needed and does not work for preventing or treating these diseases.

Medical industry obstructionism

The medical industry's lobbying groups, such as the American Cancer Society and the American Heart Association, have historically been resistant to educating the public about diet. They stand firmly on a platform built by drug money. They consistently resist and label any therapy as "quackery" that doesn't fit into the industrial box.

The medical-industrial complex complains about the public's lack of knowledge on medical issues. For instance, they blame patients for demanding antibiotics when they're not necessary. But who if not the medical community should have been doing the educating? And whose interest does it serve to have an under-educated public blindly following the dictates of MDs? If the industry had put as much money into educating the public about basic health-care issues as they have fighting "unconventional" nutritional therapies, we would have a healthier population.

Food industry advertising

Not surprisingly, many people are overwhelmed and taken in by the multi-billion dollar advertising campaigns that are waged by the processed-food industry. Radio, TV, billboards, sports stadiums and schools are dominated by advertising for "fun" foods that promise to make your life better. An interesting legal twist (twist as in screwing you) is that a food corporation cannot have their "free speech" to advertise denied, but you and I can be sued for saying "Ronald McDonald is no friend of sick children."

Misinformation spread by the media

Most science reporters rely on press releases supplied by researchers and corporations with a vested interest in their research being the next big thing. Does a week pass by without a story appearing about a huge drug breakthrough in some disease's treatment?

The cancer industry is especially good at this. They are continually promising the next magic bullet. What we get instead is trillions of dollars in tax money being spent on dead-end therapies. Few media empires give much time to the less flashy story of environmental toxins that induce cancers. They claim they're responding to what the public wants, not catering to corporate influence. The fact is, however, that most media are owned by the same corporations that own the pharmaceutical industry.

Confusion and cynicism fostered by the media

The press seems to relish stories claiming that things you thought were good for you are supposedly quite deadly. "Exercise causes heart attacks." "Don't drink too much water." "Vitamin C doesn't work." "Look out for toxins in carrots."

We are inundated with the persistent message that no matter what we do, it doesn't make any difference. Isn't that exactly what the processed-food industry wants? If it doesn't seem to matter or we don't care anymore, why not drink cola for breakfast?

When you are confused or cynical, industry and ignorance win.

No choice in a land of abundance

I'm fortunate; I live in Seattle where there is a strong community of farmers' markets, organic food co-ops, and health-oriented restaurants. However, I've traveled from coast to coast and have seen that most cities and towns have far fewer resources. I'm amused when I'm traveling and am asked if I want white or dark toast - the "dark" not referring to whole, but to added coloring.

Even in Seattle, there are times when you're stuck in a situation where your only source of "food" is the local convenience store. We live in a land of abundance. We can buy a lot of stuff for little money, but it is sometimes difficult to find value. It's no wonder that so many people are over-fed but under-nourished.

You're not stupid, it's the system

You may have been eating poorly, but you're not stupid. You have not been given the all the facts. The medical professionals you trusted didn't know any better. Vested interests have done their best to keep you ignorant. Mass advertising has worked. Don't blame yourself; blame the system. Better yet, change it.

Regularly eating a Variety of Whole foods will make you healthier. It also supports organic farmers and reduces pollution caused by transportation and processing of foods. By following this program you will be committing a revolutionary act aimed at making the world less polluted and healthier. You will also be a living example of intelligent eating.

Section VIII

The Three Wisdoms Join Hands

Chapter 51

Mantra for eating healthy every day

There's a lot of information and misinformation out there regarding nutrition. What I've tried to do in **Nutrition-1-2-3** is condense this information to the essential, easily applied mantra - **Regularly eat a Variety of Whole foods**.

This mantra has thousands of years of human history to back it up. It is also supported by hundreds of research studies.

The good news is that science is coming through with great answers on how, when and what to eat. Sometimes this information gets buried, or lost under garbage bags full of misinformation, usually being espoused by someone with financial interests. But the science is there. Time and again research has supported Regularly eating a Variety of Whole foods.

> The concepts are simple but the application can be difficult. The first step toward eating right is to understand the facts.

To apply the concepts, you will find yourself in revolt against the richest corporations in the world - McDonald's, Burger King, and all of the FFFs (Fat Food Franchises). But you will find yourself standing side-by-side with organic farmers. You will be resisting the financial interests of chemical industries. Every penny you decide to spend on organic food is an economic Molotov cocktail in the boardrooms of giant agribusiness, their lobbyists and the politicians they control.

You may have heard of retail therapy - buying stuff in order to feel better. Well, when you eat according to the Three Wisdoms, you are practicing Retail Revolution. You are consciously choosing health; health for yourself, your family and for the earth.

Between 1998 and 2001 the amount of money Americans spent each year on prescription drugs rose by 40 percent. During that time, the rates of all of the crippling and killing diseases – eczema, asthma, diabetes, cancer, and heart disease - also continued to rise. The number of people who died from adverse drug reactions climbed to at least 100,000 deaths each year. I'm not saying to never use drugs, but to use them in the only way they've been shown to be helpful - for emergencies. Real health comes from lifestyle changes such as reducing toxic exposures, regular exercise and a nutritious diet.

Nutrition-1-2-3 and the principles of the Three Wisdoms create a solid dietary foundation that will prevent illness, restore health and enhance your well being. They will also help you to scrutinize health claims and evaluate research reports. Lastly, by reducing agricultural and environmental damage, this program will improve the health of the planet.

Thank you for caring about yourself and the earth.

Section IX

Nibbles of helpful information

Nibble A - Body Mass Index (BMI)

To find your BMI, draw a line between your height and weight. Your BMI is where the line intersects the center scale. Male and female charts are different. A BMI above 25 is considered overweight. Over 30 is obese. BMI is not as accurate as fat percentage in estimating health.

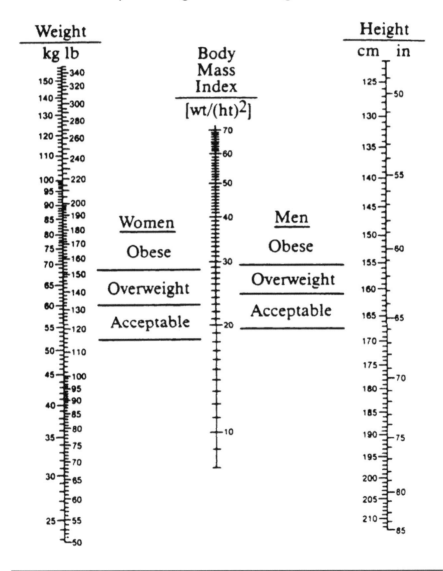

Nibble B – Waist to hip ratio

Waist to Hip Ratio Chart

Male	Female	Health Risk Based on WHR
0.95 or below	0.80 or below	Low Risk
0.96 to 1.0	0.81 to 0.85	Moderate Risk
1.0+	0.85+	High Risk

Nibble C – Protein content of common foods

(In Grams)

Grains:
Amaranth: 1 cup, 28 grams
Bagel: 1 whole, 9 g
Dinner roll: 1 roll, 2.4 g
WW Bread: 1 slice, 2.4 g
English Muffin: 1 whole, 4.5 g
Bran Flakes: 1 cup, 4.8 g
Oatmeal: 1 cup, 6 g
Sugar Frosted Flakes:1 cup, 2 g
Rice Cake: 1, 0.7 g
Rye Crisp: 1 square, 6 g
Wheat thins: 8, 1.0 g
Brown rice: 1 cup, 14.5 g
Egg noodles: 1 cup, 6.6 g
Millet: 1 cup, 22.6 g
Quinoa: 1 cup, 22 g
Popcorn: 1 cup, 1.5 g
Spaghetti (WW) 1 cup, 8.4 g

Legumes:
Black Beans: 1 cup, 15 g
Garbanzo Beans: 1 cup, 14.5 g
Lentils: 1 cup, 18.0 g
Split Peas: 1 cup, 16 g
Soybeans: 1 cup, 28.6 g

Dairy:
Cheddar Cheese: 1 oz, 7.1 g
Cottage Cheese: 1 cup, 25 g
Feta Cheese: 1 oz, 4.0 g
Jack Cheese: 1 oz, 6.9 g
Whole Milk: 1 cup, 8.0 g
Yogurt -plain: 1 cup, 8 g
Yogurt - skim: 1 cup, 13 g
Egg: 1 whole, 6.0 g
Soy milk: 1 cup, 4 – 8 g

Vegetables:
Broccoli: ½ cup, 2.3 g
Carrot: ½ cup, 0.9 g
Baked Potato: 1 large, 4.7 g
Zucchini: ½ cup, 0.6 g

Meat:
Flank Steak: 4 oz, 22 grams
Lean Ground Beef: 4 oz, 28 g
Round Steak: 4 oz, 22 g
Lamb chop: 4 oz, 25.5 g
Bacon: 3 slices, 5.8 g
Ham: 3.5 oz, 18.5 g
Roll Chicken: 2 slices, 11 g
Chicken:1 drumstick, 14 g
Chicken: 3.5 oz, 27 g
Turkey: 3.5 oz, 28 g
Turkey Roll: 2 slices, 10.3 g

Nuts and Seeds:
Almonds: 1 oz, 4.6 g; 1 cup, 26.4 g
Almond Butter: 1 Tbs, 2.4 g
Cashews: 1 oz, 4.4 g; 1 cup, 24 g
Hazelnuts: 1 oz, 3.7 g
Peanuts: 1 oz, 6.6 g
Peanut Butter: 1 T, 4 g
Pumpkin Seeds: 1 oz, 7.0; 1 cup, 40.6 g
Sunflower Seeds 1 oz, 6.5 g; 1 cup, 35 g
Sesame Butter (Tahini): 1 Tbs, 2.6 g
Walnuts: 1 oz, 4.1 g ; 1 cup,14.8 g

Fish:
Cod: 3 oz, 19.4 g
Crab: 3 oz, 16.5 g
Halibut: 3 oz, 22.7 g
Oysters: 3 oz, 12 g
Salmon - pink: 3 oz, 16.8 g
Salmon - sockeye: 3 oz, 23.2 g
Shrimp: 3 oz, 17.8 g
Tuna in water: 1 can, 42 g

Misc:
Spirulina: 1 cup, 8.6 g
Tempeh: 100 gm, 19 g
Tofu, firm: 1/2c, 10 g

Compiled by Tom Ballad, RN, ND

Nutrition Facts

Serving Size 1 cup (85g) (3 oz.)

Servings per container 2.5

Amount per serving

Calories 45   Calories from Fat 0

	% Daily Value*
Total Fat 0g	0%
Saturated Fat 0g	0%
Cholesterol 0mg	0%
Sodium 55 mg	2%
Total Carbohydrate 10g	3%
Dietary Fiber 3g	12%
Sugars 5g	
Protein 1g	

Vitamin A 360% • Vitamin C 8% • Calcium 2% • Iron 0%

*Percent Daily Values are based on a 2,000 calorie diet. Your daily value may be higher or lower depending on your calorie needs.

	Calories:	2,000	2,500
Total Fat	Less than	65g	80g
Sat. Fat	Less than	20g	25g
Cholesterol	Less than	300mg	300mg
Sodium	Less than	2,400mg	2,400mg
Total Carbohydrate	Less than	300mg	375mg
Dietary Fiber	Less than	25g	30g

Calories per gram: Fat 9 • Carbohydrate 4 • Protein 4

Ingredients: Carrots.

Note the perfect list of ingredients: no additives, no preservatives, no coloring, and no junk!
Patient comments….

Pure Wellness Shopping List

Protein

Fish
- Bass
- Cod
- Crab
- Halibut
- Herring
- Lobster
- Mackerel
- Salmon
- Shrimp
- Tilapia
- Trout

Poultry
- Chicken
- Duck
- Game
- Turkey

Meat
- Beef
- Buffalo
- Lamb
- Pork

Dairy
- Yogurt
- Cottage cheese
- Soft cheese
  - Brie
  - Feta
  - Ricotta
- Hard Cheese
  - Bleu
  - Cheddar
  - Gouda
  - Jarlsberg
  - Mozzarella
  - Parmesan
  - Provolone
  - Swiss
- Goat
- Sheep

Beans/Peas
- Azuki
- Black
- Black-eyed
- Garbanzo
- Lentils
- Lima
- Navy
- Pinto
- Red kidney
- Soy/tofu
- Split peas

Vegetables
- Chives
- Garlic
- Leeks
- Onions
- Scallions
- Shallots
- Water chestnuts

Fruit Vegetables
- Avocados
- Bitter melon
- Chayote
- Cucumbers
- Eggplant
- Okra
- Olives
- Peppers
- Squash
- Tomatoes
- Tomatillos

Inflorescent Vegetables
- Artichokes
- Broccoli
- Cauliflower

Leaf Vegetables
- Arugula
- Brussels sprouts
- Cabbage
- Chicory
- Chinese cabbage
- Collards
- Cress
- Dandelion leaves
- Nettles
- Endive
- Lamb's lettuce
- Lettuce
- Nasturtium
- Purslane
- Radicchio
- Savoy
- Sorrel
- Spinach

Root Vegetables
- Beets
- Carrots
- Parsnips
- Radishes
- Rutabaga
- Turnips

Stalk Vegetable
- Asparagus
- Bamboo
- Celery
- Chard
- Fennel
- Kohlrabi
- **Tuber Vegetable**
- Cassava
- Jerusalem artichoke
- Jicama
- Potato
- Sweet potato
- Taro
- Yam

Fruit
- Apple
- Apricots
- Banana
- Berries
  - Acai
  - Bearberry
  - Black
  - Blue
  - Cranberry
  - Currant
  - Marionberry
  - Raspberry
  - Strawberry
- Cherries
- Figs
- Grapefruit
- Kiwi
- Kumquat
- Lemons
- Limes
- Mango
- Melons
  - Cantaloupe
  - Honeydew
  - Watermelon
- Oranges
- Papaya
- Peaches
- Pears
- Pineapple
- Plums
- Quince

Supplemental Protein
- Whey
- Rice
- Soy
- Pea
- Hemp

"I never would have believed it, but my craving for sweets has completely gone away. At my daughter's wedding, I could only eat a couple of bites of the cake. It tasted too sweet." Donna, former sweet addict.

"My anxiety is way down. I can drive now." Lindsey, who has also lost 30+ pounds.

"I've lost almost 20 pounds and my chronic sinus drainage is gone. I hope to be able to start the exercise part of the program in the spring." Don

"My MD couldn't believe that my cholesterol and blood pressure could drop that much without drugs." John, former prescription drug taker.

"My sciatic pain is gone." Julie
"I stopped using all those products when my acne cleared up." Misty

"I suffered with chronic constipation for 50 years! No one ever suggested there were alternatives to laxatives." Sandra

"My sleep is no longer a problem. God does it feel good to sleep through the night." Carol

"My energy is better than it's been in 20 years." Dorothy, 82 years old.

"I love your book. It's so well organized and easy to read." John

And numerous, *"I'm glad I don't have to take that (blood pressure, cholesterol, diabetes) pill any more. Thank you."*

And thank all of you for caring about the health of the world, Tom Ballard, RN, ND

7792644R0

Made in the USA
Charleston, SC
10 April 2011

Books by Tom Ballard

Non-Fiction
- **Pure Weight Loss; Environmental detoxification and nutritional rejuvenation for lifelong weight control**
  The future of health and weight loss

- **Nutrition-1-2-3: three proven diet wisdoms for losing weight, gaining energy, and reversing chronic disease**
  The basics of natural nutrition for shopping, eating and regaining your health through nutrition

Fiction
- **The President is Down** (Novel)
  The most powerful man in the world crashes in Central America where a beautiful peasant rescues him from rebels, soldiers, and himself.

- **The Last Quack** (Novel)
  Kate Turner, naturopathic physician, discovers that tripping over a dead body may be hazardous to her health, especially when the dead woman was researching the same medicinal mushroom.

- **Eco-Agent Man: the case of the vanishing moth** (Film Script) *Nick Chronos, undercover Ecology-Agent, battles a ruthless developer to save an endangered species.*

- **Get to Know your Duck** (Play)
  The Bland family's complacent existence is scrambled when the twins bring home a two-headed duck that keeps growing… and growing…

The rewards of naturopathic medicine – patient endorsements

"You're the only doctor I've ever seen, and I've been to dozens, who has ever treated my disease. They all just want to prescribe something for my symptoms. And I've taken all their pills and only feel worse." Donna

"I should hate you because I keep having to buy smaller clothes." Peggy, former yo-yo dieter.

"I thought my energy was fine. It's one thousand percent better now." Steve.

"My MD warned me against naturopathy…. (but)…My asthma is something I don't have to worry about any more." Kelly, whose asthma had sent her to the emergency room several times before finding naturopathy.

"I've been losing about two pounds a week… No, I'm surprised, but I'm never hungry." Rene.

"I can't believe how good my joints feel!" Carla, long-time arthritis sufferer.

"No vitamin has ever made me feel as good as this." Don, after over twenty years of being a self-described health-food nut.

"I feel like I'm breathing into areas of my lungs that have never felt air before." Susan, asthma patient.

"Every day my skin feels softer. Sometimes people don't recognize me." Lois, after having severe eczema since childhood.

"I'm so thankful to you that I didn't have to have that bowel surgery." Francine, after five years of debilitating celiac disease.

Read more comments on back cover….